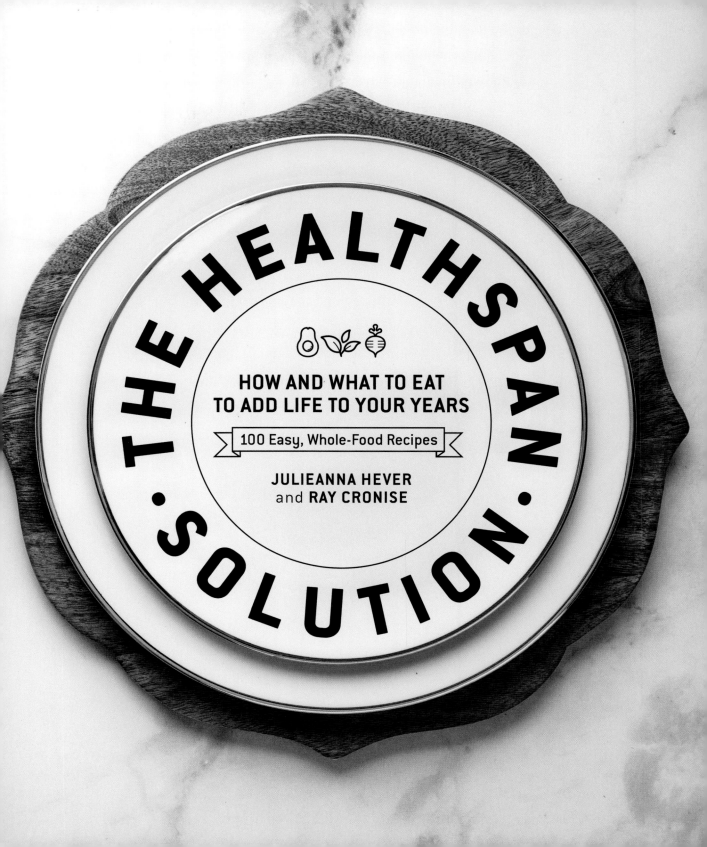

THE HEALTHSPAN

HOW AND WHAT TO EAT
TO ADD LIFE TO YOUR YEARS

100 Easy, Whole-Food Recipes

JULIEANNA HEVER
and RAY CRONISE

SOLUTION

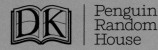

This book is dedicated to our collective plantlings: Alexia, Erin, Danner, Maya, and Benjamin. We wish you all long lives filled with love, health, and happiness, inspired by inquisitiveness and exploration, and infused with passion, independent thought, and adventure. —J.H. and R.C.

Publisher: Mike Sanders
Senior Editor: Ann Barton
Senior Designer: Jessica Lee
Art Director: William Thomas
Photographer: Kelley Schuyler
Food Stylist: Savannah Norris
Recipe Tester: Trish Malone
Proofreaders: Charles Hutchinson, Rick Kughen, Lisa Starnes
Indexer: Celia McCoy

First American Edition, 2019
Published in the United States by DK Publishing
6081 E. 82nd Street, Indianapolis, Indiana 46250
Copyright © 2019 by Raymond J. Cronise and Julieanna Hever

19 20 21 22 23   10 9 8 7 6 5 4 3 2 1
001-316435-JAN2020

Published in the United States by Dorling Kindersley Limited.

ISBN: 978-1-4654-9007-0

Library of Congress Catalog Number: 2019945959

Note: This publication contains the opinions and ideas of its authors. It is intended to provide helpful and informative material on the subject matter covered. It is sold with the understanding that the authors and publisher are not engaged in rendering professional services in the book. If the reader requires personal assistance or advice, a competent professional should be consulted. The authors and publisher specifically disclaim any responsibility for any liability, loss, or risk, personal or otherwise, which is incurred as a consequence, directly or indirectly, of the use and application of any of the contents of this book.

Trademarks: All terms mentioned in this book that are known to be or are suspected of being trademarks or service marks have been appropriately capitalized. Alpha Books, DK, and Penguin Random House LLC cannot attest to the accuracy of this information. Use of a term in this book should not be regarded as affecting the validity of any trademark or service mark.

DK books are available at special discounts when purchased in bulk for sales promotions, premiums, fund-raising, or educational use. For details, contact SpecialSales@dk.com.

Printed and bound in Canada

Author photos (pages 6 and 256) © Melissa Schwartz
All other images © Dorling Kindersley Limited
For further information see: www.dkimages.com

A WORLD OF IDEAS:
SEE ALL THERE IS TO KNOW

CONTENTS

INTRODUCTION

Over the last decade, so much has changed that may impact our view of health and longevity. For millennia, people from all walks of life strived to get the minimum to survive. Our biology adapted to a world of scarcity, and humans did so well that we are able to successfully inhabit a wide range of environments. We've even had humans living in space continuously aboard the International Space Station since November 2, 2000. The acceleration in our engineering and agricultural prowess during the twentieth century resulted in our mastery of the environment. This was bolstered by infectious disease control, antibiotics, and emergency medicine. Since the advent of refrigeration and affordable worldwide transportation, our access to food has immeasurably changed the world, and that access is probably second in importance to the time when our ancestors mastered cooking. It seems that above all else, our unique ability to cook was one of the most important steps in our environmental mastery and led to the widespread flourishing of our species.[1]

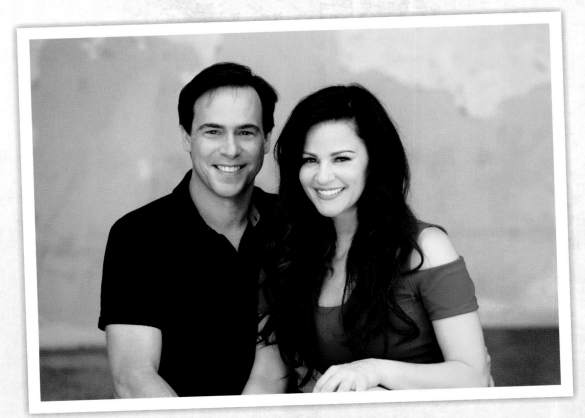

In the nineteenth century, cookbooks targeted at common households were becoming more popular. Many included information beyond cooking instructions, such as why we should or shouldn't eat certain food, appropriate table manners, and even ways to combat social injustices. As food became more economically available, it began to have an increasing influence on society beyond basic nourishment. Food is now so cheap and plentiful that there are people who are somewhat anti-cooking and promote eating only raw food. This luxury of abundance is likely what gave rise to our current society, which is chronically overnourished. That is one message we hope this cookbook will make clear to you.

Over the past decade, we (Julieanna and Ray) have collectively researched diet and nutrition in the lab, scoured the scientific literature, and practically applied our findings in our work with hundreds of clients. Over the last few years, our individual messages converged to one unified idea. We thought it was more important to include a little history and science in the limited pages we had to introduce that idea than to teach you how to sauté or organize your pantry. There are no meal plans. We aren't here to villainize any food or promote something to superfood status. We aren't anti-carb, anti-fat, or pro-artichoke. We don't care where you get your protein, and not only that, we don't even use that label as a salient description of food. You won't find the typical meal categories of breakfast, lunch, snack, and dinner in this book; there are no desserts. This is the food we love to eat. We will present a growing body of evidence that it may be the most enjoyable way to implement the only dietary intervention that has extended an organism's life.

We're grateful for our publisher allowing us to travel so far off the well-worn cookbook path of *how* to explore the less-considered passages of *why*. Instead of a lifeless, single-font listing of ingredients and instructions in the back of an academic tome, we are excited by the appetizing photography to bolster the fascinating history and science. It may be a lot to take in for one read, but we hope you'll litter the cooking pages with stains and the front material with highlighters, dog-eared pages, and sticky notes.

The Healthspan Solution is your simple blueprint for how and what to eat to deliciously optimize your health, sustainably manage your weight, and to not just live longer, but to live longer with vitality, clarity, and intention. Thank you for taking this healthspan journey with us and we hope you'll keep eating right.

CHAPTER 1

OUR BROKEN PLATE

OUR HEALTHCARE CRISIS AND HOW WE ENDED UP HERE

You're not going to live forever eating carrots. Our message isn't one of immortality. We also want to steer clear of food ideology or diet hacks. For more than a decade, both of us have spent time digging through the literature, working with clients, collaborating with other researchers, and speaking around the world. We both also love to eat. At times, we both felt frustrated from the seemingly ever-evolving sugar versus fat conundrums. There's far more to delve into than can be covered in the introductory chapters of a cookbook, but we'd like to share a simple framework that might be useful when considering the disparate food facts collected along the way: you're not broken; more likely it's *our broken plate*. Whatever your age, size, or athletic ability, most of the apparent contradictions about food are rooted in how we organize, study, and sell it—not broken physiology.

> **" You're not broken; more likely it's *our broken plate.* "**

In nature, there are no contradictions. The world is what it is, but the way we interpret our observations of the world can often be rife with apparent contradictions. Is a potato a carb? Where do we get protein? Is a tomato a vegetable or fruit? We love to catalog and organize things because it helps simplify a world that is too complex for anyone to fully comprehend. In that process, we must compress all of these observations into an easier-to-digest view—and in that compression, we toss out lots of data. Over the last two to three centuries, we've come to think of food in a fundamentally different way than humans did during the millennia that our ancestors have walked the earth.

In summary, our view of food changed dramatically once we moved to a late eighteenth-century, metabolism-centric, food-body model of Antoine Lavosier. While people likely always saw food as fuel, his discovery and assertion that respiration and combustion are identical chemical processes equated the vital force of life to an inanimate flame. This meant that a candle burning wax (fat) as fuel while consuming oxygen and producing carbon dioxide, water, heat, and light, was the same process as the so-called inner heat in humans and animals. This was a radical shift in how people conceptualized food, in that life became less mystical and more mechanical.

The fathers of nutritional science, Justus von Liebig, Carl von Voit, and Max Rubner, moved food in three different ways in the nineteenth century. First, they discovered crop rotation and fertilization, which allowed unprecedented agricultural productivity. Next, they cataloged the fuel components of food, which we now know as proteins, carbohydrates, fats, and alcohol, and could measure the metabolic impacts in laboratories. Finally, they introduced the concept of a dietary Calorie (actually a kilocalorie, or 1,000 calories) such that exacting measurement of fuel input and output could be studied. We began the twentieth century with von Liebig's notion of "protein plus fuel" conceptualization of food—the idea that the protein components of food are the tissue-forming elements of life and the fats and carbohydrates fuel the process.

COOKING UP SALES

These history and science lessons may seem somewhat out of step with a cookbook, but the idea dates back to a cookbook written by Eliza Acton and published in London in 1858, only 15 years after Justus von Liebig had introduced this new "protein plus fuel" framework for food. This book was one of the first cookbooks written for Britain's middle class and remained in print for over 50 years. Titles were particularly flavorful and long at that time, and this title might shed light on our interest in this particular edition, *Modern Cookery, For Private Families, Reduced to a System of Easy Practice, In a Series of Carefully Tested Receipts, In Which the Principles of Baron Liebig and Other Eminent Writers Have Been as Much as Possible Applied and Explained*. Our editors would have fired us had we turned in such a title for this book. Beyond the wordiness, we shouldn't overlook the significance of this cookbook, because it was integrating—for the first time—cutting edge science with cookery and pushing that information out to the everyday population. What she writes in the preface is both prophetic and chilling:

I have zealously endeavoured to ascertain, and to place clearly before my readers, the most rational and healthful methods of preparing those simple and essential kinds of nourishment which form the staple of our common daily fare; and have occupied myself but little with the elegant superfluities or luxurious novelties with which I might perhaps more attractively, though not more usefully, have filled my pages. Should some persons feel disappointed at the plan I have pursued, and regret the omissions which they may discover, I would remind them, that the fashionable dishes of the day may at all times be procured from an able confectioner; and that part of the space which I might have allotted to them is, I hope and believe, better occupied by the subjects, homely as they are, to which I have devoted it—that is to say, to ample directions for dressing vegetables, and for making what cannot be purchased in this country unadulterated bread of the most undeniably wholesome quality; and those refreshing and finely-flavoured varieties of preserved fruit which are so conducive to health when judiciously taken, and for which in illness there is often such a vain and feverish craving when no household stores of them can be commanded.

Merely to please the eye by such fanciful and elaborate decorations as distinguish many modern dinners, or to flatter the palate by the production of new and enticing dainties, ought not to be the principal aim, at least, of any work on cookery. "Eat,— *to live*" should be the motto, by the spirit of which all writers upon it should be guided.[1]

> **" ...not only does science impact food marketing, but the marketing of food also impacts science. "**

It's fascinating that the first few pages of a mid-nineteenth century cookbook has described the same issues that face us 160 years later, namely: decadent versus simple food, eating out versus at home, and designing recipes primarily for health.

Liebig developed and widely promoted a method to extract what he believed to be the health-beneficial elements of meat and Eliza Acton in part captured this cold-extract processing for cooking so anyone could do this at home. Liebig began selling LEMCO Meat Extract in 1847, and by the early twentieth century, his Oxo brand was introduced, which is still sold today. This is the origin of beef bouillon, and while it didn't increase healthfulness of food, it did well in terms of sales. The rows of bone broth on market shelves today are driven by much the same sort of good-story, nostalgic reflection combined with our overall societal drive to prioritize food sales and palate entertainment over the role of eating for health.

We should recognize that these were best-guess food practices at the time. We'll discuss the umami contribution these early meat extracts likely played in food preparation and some of the implications for healthspan; however, in the larger context, these science-commercial intersections have slowly redefined how we think about and organize food. Even researchers and healthcare professionals are subject to the pervasive influence of food marketing. It's important to keep in mind that not only does science impact food marketing, but the marketing of food also impacts science.

COUNTING CALORIES

American researchers Wilbur Olin Atwater and Graham Lusk, both students of von Voit, ushered in the twentieth century through widespread popularization of both calories and macronutrient food organization of nutrition and metabolism. As the original scientist for the United States Department of Agriculture (USDA), Atwater popularized the calorie among the wider population beginning with his first article in the July 1887 issue of *New Century Monthly Magazine*.[2] He began issuing a series of bulletins on food and diet that continued until his death in 1907. A year before his death, Yale Nutritional Scientist Graham Lusk introduced the first nutrition textbook. Together, they brought a completely new perspective to food. The role of food in health, for example, its relationship to diabetes and cardiovascular disease, was systematically studied in relationship to the fundamental nutritional components of food. At the same time, the USDA's main focus was on the economy of food production.

Because food was economically scarce, much of Atwater's work was centered on finding the best nutrition for the least cost, what he called the "nutritive value of food." Atwater simultaneously promoted food for both its role in health and the economic prosperity to farmers across the United States who were funding the research efforts. His early attention to the nutritive value of food and solving the economics of feeding the poor is evident when in 1894 he writes,

> The most striking fact brought out by all these calculations is the difference between the animal and vegetable foods in the actual cost of nutriment. Meats, fish, poultry, and the like are expensive, while flour and potatoes are cheap food. The reason of this is simple. The animal foods are made from vegetable products. Making meat from grass or grain is costly. An acre of land will produce a given number of bushels of wheat, but when the grass or grain which the same land would produce is converted to meat it makes much less food than the wheat.[3]

Atwater was keenly aware that it made more economic sense to feed the crops directly to people rather than feed the crops to livestock and then feed the animals to people. This is still true today. More than 2,400 foods were analyzed for their macronutrient compositional makeup in over one hundred agricultural experiment stations across the United

"...by 2011, the worldwide number of overnourished outnumbered undernourished for the first time in history."

States and in Europe.[4] Food groups were introduced, and by 1916, the USDA School Lunch Program sought to both help address childhood malnutrition, which was primarily economically based, and to promote agricultural products to homemakers.[5] Food production and sales were tools of foreign policy during World War I and the US exported food around the world. By the 1920s, the economy of food was in full swing, and with the exception of the depression and wars, the percentage of household income spent on food has dropped over the last century from nearly 50 percent to less than 10 percent. It's staggering to ponder that we struggled for centuries to get *enough* and, according to the World Health Organization, by 2011, the worldwide number of overnourished outnumbered undernourished for the first time in history. Obesity is now a symptom of poverty.

Today, it's almost cliché to mock food labels and advertisements. In 1974, Donald S. McLaren wrote an article for the esteemed medical journal, *The Lancet*, entitled "The Great Protein Fiasco." This article chronicles how malnutrition in Africa in the 1930s was economically exploited to create a perceived nutritional protein deficiency crisis. As we write this, protein is all the rage again on food labels. Yet, as we will discuss, trying to define food by major macronutrient concentrations, like protein, not only doesn't describe metabolically similar foods, but as importantly, protein restriction without malnutrition is one of

"...protein restriction without malnutrition is one of the few nutritional interventions that has been shown to extend the life of a model organism, from yeast to primates."

the few nutritional interventions that has been shown to extend the life of a model organism, from yeast to primates. The silver lining, or should we say, cherry on top, is that many people now live in a *luxus* environment that doesn't require scavenging and hunting for food. We have even conquered the seasons and have plentiful supplies of vegetables, fruits, whole grains, legumes, mushrooms, nuts, seeds, herbs, and spices year-round. We aren't implying that one can't be overnourished on this diet, particularly if adulterants such as sugar, flour, salt, and oil are used indiscriminately. On the contrary, if one can make adjustments that may go against current social norms, this diet may be the most enjoyable way to implement the *less is more* strategy that longevity and healthspan research over the last century has uncovered. Success here isn't hampered by access to the right food, but rather on mitigating social pressures that seem to dominate our plates.

SURVIVING IN A SOCIETY CENTERED AROUND EATING

We are now living in a society of one meal that takes breaks to work and sleep. Everything revolves around food—vacations, business, holidays, religious events, movies, and even funerals. Imagine for just a moment that you invited some of your friends over to watch a movie or a game and didn't have anything to eat or drink. They could grab some water if they were thirsty, but you would serve no snacks, meals, or desserts. The idea seems uncomfortable to most people.

Although we get together to do many things, food is the universal social lubricant. Of course, our goal writing a cookbook isn't to denigrate these societal norms, but rather to point out that food access and social pressure to eat are two of the primary reasons why the overnourished outnumber the undernourished worldwide. When people take religious or ideological stances on eating certain foods, it can often cause great conflict with friends and family, or it may create social isolation. We aren't completely free to teach our children to eat because billions of dollars are spent promoting food to them, and they are subject to social pressures from friends at school, just as adults experience social pressures at a business lunch or social gathering. Not only can eating differently cause friction, many people believe they are experts, merely because they eat.

Reading any article, blog, or book, including this one, isn't the final word on food. It is a complex subject with lots of nuance. There are many reasons performing studies is difficult, but among the more important ones is that food is an integral part of human-human and human-animal socialization. Nutritionally induced chronic disease happens over decades, and that spans so much of human social life. It's impractical to feed a human a precisely controlled diet for more than a couple of months. Even primate feeding studies that began in the late 1980s to mid-90s have taken more than four decades to complete. Where we can see direct social influence on food is with our pets. Advertisers place food flavors on labels for the humans that purchase the food; it's not for a starving cat or dog. Our pets succumb to the same diseases of overnutrition as humans: cancers, diabetes, cardiovascular disease, and autoimmune disorders.

We socialize pets with food, and a big reason you are part of their social world is because you feed them. There can be no doubt that both you and your pet get joy from the table scraps or treats at least one of you knows isn't the best long-term health choice, but we do it anyway. Likewise, we make exception after exception when it comes to our own diets and eating with others. Breaking this cycle is difficult as someone will always offer the extreme retort, "Live a little; you're going to die of something." This might be

> "Deprivation in a culinary sense is tied more to habit than survival, but creating new habits does take focus and time."

true and completely irrelevant to our individual journeys.

Equally important is that all food is habit, and when one travels the world, decadent foods take on many different definitions. If favorite foods are decadent and malleable, one of your new favorite foods might be in this book—many of our favorite recipes certainly are here. Once you've adapted to a new food habit, eating this way feels no more depriving than a nonsmoker feels deprived of cigarettes. Deprivation in a culinary sense is tied more to habit than survival, but creating new habits does take focus and time.

A NEW NORMAL

We teach our lifestyle transformation clients that until the new diet is equally convenient, familiar, and enjoyable as the old, you don't have a choice; one or more of these will likely dominate your plate. This cookbook is a launching platform to a new lifestyle. Some of the recipes are decadent, and some of them are quite ordinary. What will likely be true for everyone is that it will take some time to master the 8 to 10 recipes that you can shop for, cook, and serve without a list or directions. You'll need to be able to scan the pantry or refrigerator and find an enjoyable on-the-go meal. It will take some time to figure out a best strategy at restaurants or on vacations.

There's simply no way to escape social interaction surrounding food, but we don't need to escape it, as it is manageable no matter where you are. Most of us live with other people and they may or may

"There's no reason you can't make a change—and it need not disrupt the lives of your friends, family, and colleagues around you."

not share your desire to make a lifestyle change. That's okay; be a lighthouse, not a tugboat. While it might seem contrary, the more people you involve in a lifestyle transformation, the more difficult it often is to make the change. Since you can't be a total isolationist, you'll typically need to strike a balance, but don't let that balance become a path to mediocre moderation. There's no reason you can't make a change—and it need not disrupt the lives of your friends, family, and colleagues around you.

We no longer label meals as breakfast, lunch, and dinner except on the rare occasion that these meal monikers are needed to open the discussion. Does it matter what time of day you "break fast" or what that meal's flavor palate is? These labels are great for restaurants. It helps them plan what to put on the menu at a particular time of day, but these time–of–day food palate rules are arbitrary and limiting. It's not necessary to eat on 21 to 42 separate occasions each week. Twenty-four centuries ago Hippocrates suggested,

> We must consider, also, in which cases food is to be given once or twice a day, in greater or smaller quantities, and at intervals. Something must be conceded to habit, to season, to country and to age.[6]

In one of Atwater's first USDA bulletins on food, he wrote,

> In our actual practice of eating, we are apt to be influenced too much by taste, that is, by the dictates of the palate; we are prone to let natural instinct be overruled by acquired appetite. We need to observe our diet and regulate appetite by reason. In doing this we may be greatly aided by the knowledge of what our food contains and how it serves its purpose in nutrition.[7]

And yet, we know more about nutrition than any time in human history and, for the first time, we have managed to achieve a decline in health and a rise in early death through excesses of diet on a worldwide scale. Corpulence and diseases of affluence were once the domain of the wealthy, and they are now more prevalent in cases of poverty. Billions of dollars are spent competing for your palate. Rather than wander off on discussions of addictive foods, corporate conspiracies, or hidden government agendas, let's just agree that no one should tell you what or when to swallow. It's completely up to you. Equally important, you probably shouldn't spend a lot of time telling other people what to swallow.

Our request, as you begin to explore your own palate and work on your new favorite foods, is to focus the curiosity inward. It's your turn to be an example, a healthspan lighthouse, and let your actions shine. If you stick to it, they might even light the way for others around you.

We'll say it again, chances are high that *you're not broken*. Finding your new normal may take a while. Flavors will change and new favorite foods will blossom with time. What's surprising is how quickly the old favorite foods are displaced. You'll likely still enjoy many of them, because they are anchored to some emotional event of your life, like that old favorite song, but you won't need to plate them on repeat.

"It's your turn to be an example, a healthspan lighthouse, and let your actions shine."

We teach our clients to use "rare and appropriate" (R&A) in place of cheat days. R&A is based on people and places, not the time between events. When people commit to a cheat day every week or month, the timing often drives the cheat. With R&A, you might find yourself in a small temple in China with a local who's offering not only an impassioned piece of their culture, but something you likely won't experience again. Treasure these moments and deviate. If every meal is a celebration, no meals are celebrations. Moderation is a worn path to living with old habits and often hides all the amazing foods and flavors you've yet to appreciate. Before we get into the decadent, delicious deviations, let's take a look at the scientific underpinnings of the healthspan solution.

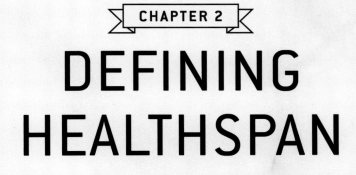

CHAPTER 2

DEFINING HEALTHSPAN

WHAT IS HEALTHSPAN?

With a little food history, economics, and sociology out of the way, we begin to see that many cultural norms surrounding eating may be based on fragile foundations. Let's move into some new ideas that may provide a better framework for you to organize food. When we discuss how long we live, there are a lot of statistical metrics one could use—absolute years alive, average age, median age, etc. According to the 2016 health-adjusted life expectancy report from the World Health Organization (WHO), lifespan for both sexes combined ranges from 83.7 years in Japan to 50.1 years in Sierra Leone.[1] After correcting for severe economic conditions, substandard healthcare, and political strife, it's reasonable to pick 80 years overall. As of now, you're going to die,

and we can't change that (yet). How and when you die does have some flexibility. Are you going to fall asleep and not wake up one day, or will you spend the last five years battling a chronic disease, in and out of a hospital? What will be the quality of your life from right now until you become a plus or a minus on the average lifespan statistics? That's what we want to focus on when discussing healthspan. Whereas *lifespan* refers to the total number of years alive, *healthspan* focuses on how many living years one remains healthy and free of disease or dysfunction.

Specifically, we define healthspan as the period of life spent in good health, free from chronic diseases and disabilities of aging. It takes about 15 years to reach reproductive age, followed by 15 to 20 years of reproductive prime, and finally,

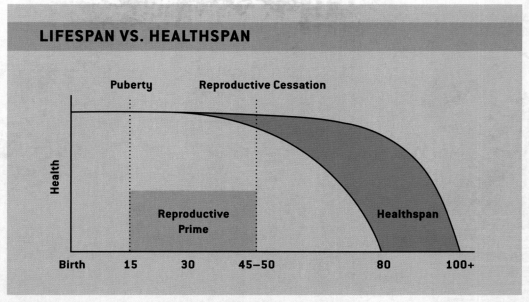

LIFESPAN VS. HEALTHSPAN

Puberty — Reproductive Cessation

Health

Reproductive Prime

Healthspan

Birth — 15 — 30 — 45–50 — 80 — 100+

Whereas "lifespan" refers to the total number of years alive, "healthspan" focuses on how many living years one remains healthy and free of disease or dysfunction.

> **"It may be that there is a trade-off between how we live during our younger years and how rapidly we age when we are older."**

an additional 15 years to raise our youngest offspring. At around 45 to 50 years of age, evolution is done with us. Those ancestral diets everyone is quick to point to, such as paleo, may well help you reach reproductive age and successfully have offspring, but they don't necessarily mitigate age-related disease after your reproductive prime is over. It's possible we need a different eating strategy to maximize each of these periods. It may be that there is a trade-off between how we live during our younger years and how rapidly we age when we are older.

WHAT SHOULD WE EAT?

All this bleak talk of death, mortality, and physical demise isn't an attempt to drive complacency. Rather, we'd like to open your mind to the possibility that eating habits could dramatically change your quality of life, particularly during the second half, after your reproductive prime. Think about healthspan in a different way: a century ago, we spent a larger percentage of our life expectancy in good health, but of course, our lives were shorter. Over the last century, through advances in primary access to food, infectious diseases, emergency medicine,

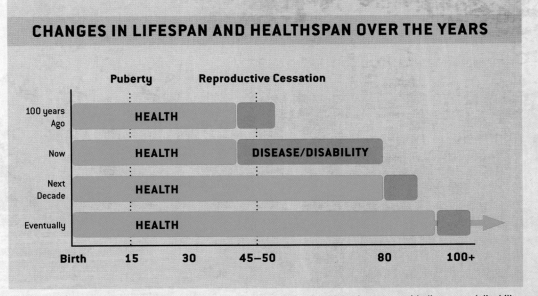

CHANGES IN LIFESPAN AND HEALTHSPAN OVER THE YEARS

The evolution of healthspan throughout lifespan, aiming to reduce time spent with disease and disability.

> **"Food is probably the single lifestyle modification anyone can make to significantly increase healthspan and add quality years of enjoyable life to the end."**

and sanitation, many have extended the period of their lives in decline, i.e., live long and die slow. With proper diet and advances in pharmacological interventions, we can probably decrease the portion of our longer lives spent in decline, i.e., live long and die fast. There are no biological limits to suggest we can't achieve both and live even longer and healthier lives.

And this brings us back to the question, "we'll die of something anyway; why bother with diet?" People would probably not say the same thing in the ambulance on the way to the emergency room or when facing a round of chemotherapy. We'd like you to consider quality of life from a much broader standard than eating hotdogs at the game or pizza at a birthday party. No matter how enjoyable those foods may have been in your past, the enjoyment you get from them doesn't equate to the backslide in health they likely will lead to without change. We aren't asking you to choose between turkey and tofu, but rather suggesting that there is a wide range of amazing food that you may not be aware of—maybe even a new favorite food—that could have a profound impact on your health. Food is probably the single lifestyle

modification anyone can make to significantly increase healthspan and add quality years of enjoyable life to the end.

First, we'd like to spend a little time discussing the aging process to give context to how some of the various changes in diet may benefit and increase the number of healthy years in your life.

THE SCIENCE OF AGING

You're probably familiar with the outward physical changes associated with aging, but you may not be aware of some of the theoretical models of aging. The field is advancing so rapidly that there's no way to cover aging in any great detail here, but we can give one a general idea of the broader field of aging research and some foundational material for further exploration. One of the most striking things we've learned about aging, particularly in the last 20 years, is that much of the underlying biology is conserved across a wide range of organisms. That is to say that when scientists examine organisms at the cellular or genetic level, there's evidence to suggest many similarities.

The next important point is that there are certain environmental factors, for example seasonal diet and temperature, that can modulate certain aging genes. When the cell is genetically altered to delete the gene, temperature and diet no longer have any effect.

What Is Aging?

All biological organisms, from tiny, single-celled bacteria to more complex species like plants or animals, change over time. Some of these changes, such as reaching reproductive age, can be seen as beneficial; other changes, like becoming frail in life's final years, can be detrimental. This concept that living organisms change over time, from birth to death, is the most general definition of aging. We might associate aging with changes in skin, memory, or hair color. In some cases, we consider aging to be a collection of age-related diseases. One might consider a question: if we could eventually cure each disease, would we in fact cure aging? For most people, this becomes a deeply difficult question or thought. And yet, there's no single disease we may die from that anyone would automatically think we shouldn't cure because "everyone needs to die of something." Bypassing the moral and social considerations, this accumulation of age-related disease at the organism level does not capture the notion of aging at the cellular level.

A more narrow definition is known as *senescence*. This can be conceptually imagined as the programmed deterioration of a cell, eventually losing the ability to divide. For example, the new leaves appear on a tree in the spring, divide and grow through the summer, and then become senescent and eventually die through a process called *apoptosis* in the fall.[2] This programmed life cycle may, in this case, serve the larger plant in that limited sun is available during the winter months, and the risk of ice and snow collecting could reduce the overall plant survivability.

Senescence plays out in yeast cells that can produce a daughter cell every 90 minutes, but they begin to lose their ability to reproduce by the second day and die in the third. At the other end of the life cycle spectrum is the single-celled hydra, a small freshwater tubular organism that attaches to a surface and then captures prey through its medusa-looking stinging tentacles. Hydra are considered biologically immortal; they don't seem to even age or die of old age.[3][4] They are capable of regeneration when cut in half, each piece regenerating the lost half in a similar way to a plant cutting that can grow new roots to become a genetically identical plant.

Historically, there are three main evolutionary theories of aging that emerged.[5][6] *Mutation Accumulation* involves random, detrimental mutations that happen and show their effects later in life. Senescence is the result of deleterious gene mutations that accumulate in older individuals. In *Antagonistic Pleiotropy,* a gene has two or more effects, both of which may be beneficial or detrimental. Genes may offer benefits early in life, but result in a health decline later in life. *Disposable SOMA* suggests the body must budget the amount of energy available, and that creates a competitive trade-off among metabolism, reproduction, and repair.

We think of evolution in terms of the adaptations that forge our species forward—a Darwinian survival of the fittest. On the other hand, much of what we see as deleterious aging happens after

LIFESPAN INTERVENTIONS WITH MODEL ORGANISMS

	LIFESPAN INCREASE		HEALTH BENEFITS
	Dietary Restriction	**Mutations/Drugs**	**Dietary Restriction**
Yeast	3-fold	10-fold (with dietary restriction)	Extended reproductive period
Worms	2- to 3-fold	10-fold	Resistance to misexpressed toxic proteins
Flies	2-fold	60-70%	None reported
Mice	30-50%	30-50% (~100% in combination with dietary restriction)	Protection against cancer, diabetes, atherosclerosis, and cardiomyopthy, as well as autoimmune, kidney, and respiratory diseases; reduced neurodegeneration
Monkeys	Trend noted	Not Tested	Prevention of obesity; protection against diabetes, cancer, and cardiovascular disease

When scientists examine a wide range of organisms, a familiar pattern emerges, but what is even more fascinating is that there also appears to be shared genes affecting lifespan and healthspan. (Adapted from Fontana, 2010.)[78]

reproductive prime. At this point, evolution is mostly done with us. The kinds of traits that would boost reproduction early or take us completely out of the game don't matter as much to our offspring after our reproductive prime because our genes have already been let loose on the world. That puts less pressure on us after reproduction, and we see this trade-off between reproduction and maintenance in many organisms.

Aging Research

Beginning in the late 1990s, work on the genes that controlled aging in various organisms began to surge. Starting with simple organisms like yeast, and moving to more complex worms, fruit flies, mice, and eventually primates, researchers began to first identify a set of proteins that seemed to impact aging and then genes that control the production of those proteins. To everyone's surprise, and with great debate in the literature, it turned out these genes were replicated throughout biology. The good news for aging (or perhaps for staying younger) seems to be that scientists can now activate and deactivate these genes. This can serve to either slow down or speed up aging. A simple, but not completely accurate, way to think about aging is to envision it as a balance between "go-go-grow" and "live longer to reproduce when conditions are better." It's not a foreign idea for most people to realize that the struggle and stress of exercise is what results in the increased strength. As the adage says, "What doesn't kill us makes us stronger." This process is called *hormesis* and it's found entangled in many different mechanisms of aging.

Specifically, hormesis is the sweet spot of a number of internal or external stresses. Too much stress can cause damage, and too little stress is easily ignored, but at the right stress level, it turns out that our cells can, paradoxically, become more robust. Phytonutrients produced by plants may help, in part, due to a phenomenon known as *xenohormesis,* which describes benefits from ingesting protective compounds created by plants when stressed.[9] [10] [11] [12] One famous example of this is resveratrol, which is found in the skin of grapes and in red wine. Although one would need to drink a thousand bottles a day to get the therapeutic dose, it didn't stop the food marketers from seizing sales. Food marketing is a place of frequent exaggeration.

In 1935, Cornell biochemist Clive McKay reported results on feeding and growth retardation in rats. Three groups of animals were fed nutritionally equivalent food, but two of the groups received fewer overall calories. This stunted growth, but it had an interesting side effect: the rats lived nearly twice as long. The longest lived of the restricted group lived almost three times the average lifespan of the normally fed rats.[13] Now, 85 years later, the only nutritional intervention of life extension that has worked on nearly all organisms, from yeast to primates, has been dietary restriction without malnutrition. It seems that nature activates these stress-induced protective genes, perhaps to preserve us until conditions are good for reproductive success.

MOLECULAR MECHANISMS OF AGING

Packing and unpacking our genetic code is one of the problems we have with aging. Our cells must unwind sections of a complex DNA sequence, and that becomes problematic as we age. If you want an introduction to underlying mechanisms for the most promising dietary and pharmacological healthspan interventions, there's no way to avoid an alphabet stew of biomolecules and molecular pathways: NAD+, mTOR, sirtuins, AMPK, IGF-1, GH, NMN, etc. We can't cover them in much detail, but since they're being discussed on many podcasts, blogs, and social media, perhaps we can at least frame them conceptually.

Our Genetic Blueprints

We start as a single fertilized egg, inheriting DNA from both parents. As that egg divides and grows, the many cells branch off into specialized functions: some become the retina cells in our eyes, while others mature into our liver cells. Other than red blood cells, the DNA of each cell in your body has the blueprint for every other cell in your body. These long chains of instructions are our recipes for life.

In response to certain environmental conditions or biological time clocks, genes can be activated or repressed through many different mechanisms. When a certain gene needs to be utilized in day-to-day cellular housekeeping, it must be unpacked, read, and then put back in place. Scientists once hypothesized that random breaks and repairs in the DNA caused a scrambled damage that accumulated over one's life to an untenable genetic mess. Stringing the bits back together in the correct order seemed impossible. Today, it's widely believed that the modifications more or less impact how the genes are put away.

It's important to note that the pathways we'll discuss here are at the cellular or subcellular level, whereas we often talk about diseases associated with aging on a body subsystem or organ level (e.g., cardiovascular disease, breast cancer, or diabetes). Each time a cell needs to create a protein, it involves unpacking a portion of our DNA blueprint that contains the necessary information and repacking it when the process is complete. Of the 30 trillion cells in the human body, about 5 trillion have DNA. The DNA of each nucleus would be about 2 meters long if it was stretched out.[14][15] That's 10 billion kilometers of DNA if all your DNA was stretched out end to end. To put this packing problem in perspective, our solar system is about 9 billion kilometers in diameter, so stretched out, this genetic material is wider than our entire solar system.

Aging Over a Lifetime

If we consider these general phases of life—pre-reproductive age, reproductive prime, and post-reproductive prime—it's likely that biological priorities and needs change over time. Simply eating to go-go-grow throughout one's entire life might appear to be the best solution because we see people grow frail as they age. It may be true that the types of diet and activity critically important to maximize reproduction earlier in life are different than the ones we need later in life, when reproductive prime is behind us. Perhaps a life of chronic overnutrition and Olympic-level training may not be the best way to age healthfully. While diet and activity are critical components of a long life, the only

" While diet and activity are critical components of a long life, the only way we've lengthened an organism's life using nutrition is through dietary restriction without malnutrition. **"**

way we've lengthened an organism's life using nutrition is through dietary restriction without malnutrition.

Why do our systems thrive when we're young but seem to fail as we get older? The answer is increasingly focused on four genetic pathways that appear to regulate longevity: mTOR, sirtuins, AMPK, and IGF-1/GH. Let's briefly discuss these longevity pathways.

mTOR

The mechanistic (mammalian) target of rapamycin (mTOR) is a cellular signaling pathway that serves as a central regulator for cell growth, metabolism, and reproduction. Rapamycin was discovered and named in the 1960s from a bacterium in the soil on Easter Island, which locals call Rapa Nui, and it exhibited antifungal properties. The discovery of these pathway targets was a result of trying to understand its immunosuppressant and anticancer properties. Abnormal activation of mTOR contributes to many age-related chronic diseases. This pathway controls many processes that use or generate large amounts of energy and nutrients.

When mTOR signaling is defective, it can initiate numerous negative events, such as processes associated with certain cancers. For example, the dietarily essential amino acid, methionine, is known to activate mTOR and is critical in the growth of certain cancers as found in breast, colon, kidney, lung, etc. tumor cells.[16] [17] [18] Place healthy breast tissue cells in a petri dish and starve them of methionine and they survive, but breast cancer tumor cells die when starved of methionine. Methionine is highest in animal-sourced foods. Some of the benefits of dietary restriction of food may be due to the restriction of methionine and other amino acids that ultimately suppress the mTOR pathway to aging.

Sirtuins

The sirtuins are a family of seven proteins that play a critical role in aging by regulating cellular health.[19] A little background is needed for sirtuin function to be more easily understood. We'll discuss protein more specifically later, but here we are addressing individual proteins, not using "protein" in a dietary sense as a food group. Each different protein your body has a specific function. A more accurate concept of protein is similar to the use of the word *metal,* which doesn't describe with specificity the various materials of gold, silver, stainless steel, iron, brass, and copper. In this more accurate use of the term for the individual cellular proteins, they aren't a food substance to ingest, but rather something every cell in your body synthesizes. The starting material used by the cells to synthesize required proteins comes from breaking down ingested dietary protein into its components.

DNA, that long string of genes that is your blueprint for life, is how our cells store the instructions for building over 20,000 *unique proteins*—and some scientists think there are many more.[20] In order to stuff a 2-meter-long DNA strand into a tiny cell nucleus, it needs to be tightly wound and packed. It's wrapped around a cluster of eight *histones*, a tiny protein spool, to form what looks like beads on a string. These little clusters of histones with DNA wrapped around them are called *nucleosomes,* and they control access to certain regions of the DNA. Nucleosomes, in turn, are coiled, the resulting strand is subsequently coiled again, and it's finally tightly packed into a chromosome. When our bodies need a specific protein for a job—for example, the protein insulin—that specific bit of DNA blueprint needs to be unpacked, copied, and then put back in place.

Proteins form the basis for every structure and function in all living organisms (enzymes, fibers, hormones, antibodies, etc.). Like the word *metal,* the word *protein* doesn't describe a single substance. Protein sequences can be imagined like the letters, words, sentences, and paragraphs of this book. While the English language uses 26 repeating letters for words, proteins use 20 repeating animo acid units.

The DNA instructions must be used to "print" various proteins on demand, but they're wound up tightly in the cell nucleus. Packing and unpacking our genes, each a blueprint for a unique protein, requires that a specific portion of the DNA is accessible for protein replication. This is accomplished by flagging the DNA and histones with small side-group molecules that cause the nucleosomes to bind tightly to repress or loosen up to expose and express the gene.

These small side-group molecules, or methyl groups and acetyl groups, cause portions of the DNA sequence, specific genes, to be hidden or accessible.

This temporary DNA modification is called an *epigenetic modification*. These kinds of modifications to the histones don't alter the DNA sequence, but they do alter how your genes are read. Further, these modifications can be transferred to a new cell during cell division and even inherited. Methyl groups pack up the genes, and acetyl groups loosen up the bonds and unpack the genes. Of the seven sirtuins in the cell, three are in the nucleus, three are in the mitochondria (or cellular power plant), and the last one is in the cytoplasm. The basic role of sirtuin proteins is to remove acetyl groups, which allows the gene and DNA to become tightly packed again. This is equivalent to genetic housecleaning, and the sirtuins act somewhat as resets for the cell. Each of the seven sirtuins has specific functions. We know for example SIRT1 is involved in healthspan pathways, and it exists in a wide range of organisms.

In the mid-1990s, researchers at MIT saw that when they deleted certain sirtuin genes, yeast had reduced reproductive capability, and when sirtuin genes were overexpressed (i.e., extra copies), the yeast lived longer and increased reproduction.[21] [22] The sirtuins are involved in many pathways related to managing cellular energy and, as such, are likely part of the mechanisms that respond to the outside environment—light, temperature, and food. There are a host of phytonutrients,

> **"A whole-food, plant-based diet is likely one of the easiest ways to naturally implement dietary restriction without malnutrition or deprivation and take advantage of nature's healthspan protective pathways."**

such as resveratrol and quercetin, that activate the sirtuin pathways, and researchers hypothesize that these are environmental stress-signaling molecules. This pathway may be much more important than sirtuins' roles as antioxidants or antibiotics for the plant's protection.[23]

Recent research is increasingly converging to recognize that these molecules are the accelerators for healthspan, but the fuel is a coenzyme, nicotinamide adenine dinucleotide (NAD^+), and some of its biomolecular precursors, such as nicotinamide riboside (NR) and nicotinamide mononucleotide (NMN).[24] [25] [26] [27] The level of NAD^+ falls in our cells as we age, and it's critically important to have both the sirtuin activating compound (STAC) and the co-enzyme to activate the sirtuin proteins. A whole-food, plant-based diet is likely one of the easiest ways to naturally implement dietary restriction without malnutrition or deprivation and take advantage of nature's healthspan protective pathways.

AMPK

Adenosine monophosphate–activated protein kinase (AMPK) is involved in regulating energy. AMPK is a cellular energy sensor and regulates the ways our bodies use and regulate lipid (fat) and glucose metabolism in response to nutrient intakes and cellular energy stores. AMPK is present in higher levels when we are younger and may help to protect us against conditions such as obesity and glucoregulatory issues. When AMPK is activated, protein and fat synthesis are inhibited and fat oxidation is increased. AMPK activations seems to decrease as we get older, which can lead to weight gain and accelerated aging. Like sirtuins, AMPK is activated by metformin, resveratrol, quercetin, and other similar molecules found particularly in vegetables and fruits. They can also be taken directly as dietary supplements, as we've seen in the case of STACs with the sirtuin pathways. It's important to note that the AMPK, sirtuin, and mTOR pathways are very interrelated and play critical roles, both together and separately, in healthspan and longevity.

IGF-1 and GH

Insulin-like growth factor 1 (IGF-1) and growth hormone (GH) are interrelated with TOR and AMPK. IGF-1 is regulated by GH and produced by the liver in mammals. GH is secreted by the pituitary gland, and animals with decreased GH levels also have decreased circulating IGF-1. Insulin signaling is mostly involved in nutrient regulation, whereas IGF-1 regulates growth. This makes for a complex balancing act. When we are younger, we want to encourage growth, and, as one might expect, hormonally active milk proteins (whey and casein) induce rapid growth in calves. Interestingly, studies have also shown that when these proteins (common in protein powders) are given to prepubertal boys, significant rises in fasting levels of IGF-1 and insulin result.[28] Casein caused a 15 percent rise in fasting IGF-1 with no change in insulin while whey caused a 21 percent rise in fasting insulin with no change in IGF-1. We've come to accept drinking milk over a lifetime as socially normal, but what are the long-term impacts for a practice that's so biologically rare?

Some researchers believe that there is good reason to limit dairy consumption.[29] [30] [31] [32] Individuals with Laron syndrome, a rare genetic condition, have a defective GH receptor and consequently don't make IGF-1.[33] [34] They are short in stature, but they have relatively long lives that are free from diabetes, cardiovascular disease, and cancers.[35] On the other hand, increased circulating levels of IGF-1 are associated with decreased longevity and increased chronic disease.[36]

Considering these four pathways as a whole, outside of their connected

> " We may need time away from the chronically fed, warm, active, and well-lighted state for metabolic housecleaning to take place. "

metabolic paths, one feature they all have in common is a response to biological stress that appears to favor longevity. When we exercise, experience brief periods of cold, and spend more time in the fasting state, the ability to reproduce falls and longevity and healthspan seems to increase. This seems to be consistent throughout biology; surprisingly, as diverse as organisms might be, the longevity metabolic pathways are similar. Some people are lucky enough to have genes that promote one or more of these pathways. Others live in cultures that have aggregated social habits, often called "Blue Zones," that exhibit increased longevity among their populations.[37] [38] [39] If you didn't get the luck of the gene draw, there is still a lot you can do to nudge healthspan in a positive direction.

THE FUTURE OF AGING RESEARCH

In 2014, Ray wrote a paper with leading Harvard biologist and longevity researcher David Sinclair and National Institutes of Health (NIH) endocrinologist and molecular biophysicist Andrew Bremer that outlined the metabolic winter hypothesis.[40] It proposes that one explanation for periods of mild cold stress and dietary restriction having a positive effect on health and longevity in a wide range of organisms might be related to a survival mechanism that co-evolved as a response to seasonal biological stresses.

Since there's no Outlook or iCal in nature, the seasons are essentially signaled by temperature, light, and food availability. In this way, metabolic winter can be characterized by periods of cool, dark, still, and food scarcity. In contrast, metabolic summer would be characterized by warm, bright, active, and food abundance. Nearly all organisms react in some way to the seasons, and these environmental cues of temperature, light, and food availability play some daily and seasonal role. Seasonal downtimes may be the metabolic equivalent of sleep for the brain. We know that sleep is crucial for the brain health, but the brain doesn't shut down when we're asleep. Instead it does a little housecleaning, consolidating memories and clearing amyloid proteins, which may accumulate as plaques in Alzheimer's disease.[41] We may need time away from the chronically fed, warm, active, and well-lighted state for metabolic housecleaning to take place. The metabolic winter paper concludes:

> Our 7-million-year evolutionary path was dominated by two seasonal challenges—calorie scarcity and mild cold stress. In the last 0.9 inches of our evolutionary mile, we solved them both. Refrigeration and transportation have fundamentally changed the food to which we have access and the environments in which we live. We also sleep less and are exposed to considerably more artificial light, particularly in the winter months. Obesity and chronic disease are seen most often in people and the animals (pets) they keep warm and overnourished. Similar to the circadian cycle and like most other living organisms, it is reasonable to believe we also respond to the seasons and carry with us the survival genes for winter. Maybe our problem is that *winter never comes.*

Wouldn't it be a shame if the only way to live longer was to starve and freeze your butt off? The good news is that increasing healthspan doesn't require deprivation. There is also a good chance that pharmacological interventions are on the way. We have evidence from a wide range of organisms that stress-induced responses can induce internal longevity mechanisms.

It's promising that our health's fate isn't etched deterministically into our genetic code. Rather, many of our genes can be activated or repressed in response to environmental stimuli, and one of the main factors in your armamentarium is food. Most longevity and healthspan research is centered on activating the fundamental mechanisms our bodies use to mitigate issues of chronic disease. The one external method that has worked throughout biology (with nearly every organism tested) is dietary restriction without malnutrition.

One place to look for clues to how we might change our diet is to consider some of the top targets for pharmacological interventions. Can we do with a diet what drug companies strive to do with a pill? In 2015, a panel of 30 top longevity scientists representing 38 research institutions worldwide concluded that the top pharmacological targets for aging were inhibition of the GH/IGF-1 axis, inhibition of the TOR -S6K pathway, regulation of certain sirtuin proteins and

" Eat less, eat less often, and when you eat, eat more of the right things. **"**

other epigenetic modifiers, inhibition of inflammation, and chronic metformin use along with protein restriction and fasting-mimicking diets.[42]

Other than chronic metformin use, the diet described in this book achieves many of these goals, at least at some level. Although pharmacological interventions will certainly be more powerful modulators of these longevity pathways, eating a diet rich in phytonutrients and fiber while restricting animal-sourced food will go a long way toward implementing healthspan pathways until more effective methods are available.

Chronic overnutrition is often easy to diagnose using only a scale. We aren't using this in the context of vanity, beauty, or fitness modeling, because many lean people will die unnecessarily early of a chronic disease. Losing weight and not gaining it are likely governed by two very different underlying physiologies. In our evolutionary past, it's far more likely our ancestors adapted to thrive through their reproductive prime in a world of scarcity, rather than in a world of excess. Today, most of us have nearly unlimited access to food, and we've been taught to avoid deficiency. Unfortunately, it's far easier to fill the dietary DVR than it is to delete old meal episodes. People often allow relatively unimportant social commitments to swallow with friends,

family, and business colleagues to overtake the short three- to-six-month period of their lives it takes to do the things that will likely delay the onset of age-related chronic disease: eat less, eat less often, and when you eat, eat more of the right things.[43]

A diet of vegetables, fruits, whole grains, legumes, mushrooms, nuts, seeds, herbs, and spices is the easiest way to implement dietary restriction without malnutrition, especially when it's done within a shorter feeding window. In time, the new normal eating habits will displace the old. The question then becomes, which habits do we lose and which should remain? With all the contradictions and disagreement surrounding food, is there anything to learn from looking at the diet of various cultures and countries? What do we know about diet? Is less more?

LESSONS FROM HEALTHY POPULATIONS

We've demonstrated that our health isn't futilely described by our genetic code. How much control do we have over how we'll age? It should be good news to learn researchers are finding more evidence that moves us past a deterministic model of aging. While we haven't yet advanced to the fountain of youth in a pill, it now appears that many elements of aging can be controlled. Evidence now strongly suggests that modifications that take place or accumulate in genes over a lifetime might be open to protection, and that could guide tools that slow, or perhaps eventually reverse, the mechanisms of aging. To what extent are modifiable behaviors, like diet, able to make an impact on healthspan?

Genes certainly play a role, and we find grandparents, parents, and offspring may inherit long lives, and these long-lived populations can occur in a wide range of cultures. Equally important is that we also find pockets of centenarians that seem to benefit from things other than genes alone. One thing that may be a little confusing is that there exists a difference in risk markers that may statistically predict an increased chance of dying early from a certain disease or condition and what might better be referred to as a collection of good lifestyle habits that statistically favor a longer life. It's a complex subject, and scientists don't completely understand yet how it all fits together. We can look at populations of centenarians for clues on what, when, and how to eat to significantly increase our healthspan success. The Mediterranean and Okinawan diets are two of the most popular diets associated with longevity.

Unwinding The Mediterranean Mayhem

As Julieanna explained in her book, *The Vegiterranean Diet*, fish, wine, and olive oil consumption weren't likely the salient features for the success with a Mediterranean diet; instead, that success is likely attributable to a collection of habits that had overall positive lifestyle impacts.[44] The Mediterranean diet is—and always has been—a whole-food, plant-based diet. The human body is magnificent in its complexity and intricacy, as are whole-plant foods and the phytonutrients they contain. The Mediterranean diet offers a combination of whole foods at its foundation, thereby supporting a synergistic approach to health. *The Vegiterranean Diet* is an overall lifestyle, not simply a diet.

Animal products comprise up to 10 percent of total calories in the Mediterranean diet, and they are saved as celebratory food for holidays, are served in condiment-sized portions when available, or are offered more sizably in rare times of abundance. And let's not forget a core tenet of this cookbook, *deliziosa cucina* (Italian for "delicious food")! Long-term compliance and persistence with a health-promoting diet is dependent upon sustainability. People like their food to taste good, and all food is habit. A Mediterranean diet, a plant-based diet, and a plant-based Mediterranean (Vegiterranean) diet offer a nearly infinite variety of inviting cuisine.

Finally, we'll see that in healthspan and longevity research, *less is more*, and historically speaking, the populations studied had less access to food as well as less processed food than their assembly line, blue-collar, U.S. counterparts. And, as we will see next with the Okinawan centenarian success, they, too, had less-is-more habits that align well with longevity and healthspan research.

Okinawans Eat, But Not Too Much

Amongst the 47 prefectures in Japan, one small island at its southern tip, Okinawa, leads the way in terms of centenarian percentage-of-population. With the highest life expectancy rankings in Japan, this population has been studied extensively.[45]

Before we dive into the food of Okinawans, let's begin with the end in mind. When researchers examine the diet of centenarians there is often a huge discrepancy between what is eaten by them, or regionally, today compared to what was eaten 100 years ago. In fact, although it's a slight decline, Okinawans have now decreased their lifespan on average compared to the overall population due to changes in their diet.[46] The longevity advantage seen and studied in Okinawa is observed only for generations born before World War II. With the distinctive change in diet, the younger generations of Okinawans are losing their longevity advantage compared to those living in mainland Japan.

One mistake that's easy to make is to project current cultural norms into the past, and when we are trying to tease out particular characteristics of a diet that may lead to increased healthspan, it's important to reach back to the diet habits from decades ago. Similar to the change in diet that's been documented over more than a half century in the Mediterranean, we've seen changes in the diet of Okinawans, too.

Okinawans are an outstanding example of a human population that has demonstrated an extension of maximum lifespan. In addition to a high prevalence of centenarians, Okinawans also have 80 percent fewer deaths due to coronary heart disease and 40 percent fewer deaths due to cancer when compared to the United States.[47] [48] Nutrition is thought to play a key role in these favorable statistics, particularly for two reasons: their tendency towards calorie restriction and the composition of the diet itself.

Hara hachi bu translates to "eat until you are eight parts full (out of ten)" and is a principle uniquely implemented in Okinawa.[49] Essentially, this means to stop when one is about 80 percent full instead of stuffing oneself. This is perhaps the most effortless way to practice calorie restriction, as the Okinawans ended up consuming approximately 11 percent fewer calories than would have been recommended for their basal metabolic rate.[45] Even better is when the food eaten is nutritionally dense, with ample fiber, satiety is simply built in, and you end up with an easy application of the life-changing health benefits associated with dietary restriction without malnutrition.

And that is precisely what the traditional Okinawan diets are based on: *nuchi gusui*, which translates to "food is medicine." Their traditional fare consisted of a high consumption of root vegetables (particularly sweet potatoes), green and yellow vegetables, legumes (mostly from soy), and other plants, many of which contain medicinal properties, such as turmeric, sea vegetables, and bitter melon. Essentially, with minimal intake of animal products (1 percent from fish, and less than 1 percent from each meat, eggs, and dairy), the traditional Okinawan diet was almost entirely whole-food and plant-based.[50] Nutritionally, this diet is low in calories and fat, especially saturated fat, and high in phytonutrients and fiber, which we will dive into in the next chapter, demonstrating the significance of these nutrients.

Okinawans represent a wonderful example of what is possible through diet. They demonstrate that dietary restriction without malnutrition seems to be the most powerful tool we have at our disposal for improving healthspan and increasing lifespan. One population that has, at times, bested the Okinawans are the California Adventists. They are the only population in the United States that consistently ranks in longevity, and they offer further evidence that an active lifestyle, increased nut and seed consumption, lower weight, and little to no animal-sourced food are all important to healthy, long lives.[51]

Compression, Conflict, and Confusion

We can't know it all. It's much too complicated. Each of us places our own compression filter on the deluge of incoming information. During this compression exercise, we toss out information, and in the process, useful information is unintentionally deleted. In those deletion voids between the complex and the understandable, beliefs—often other people's beliefs—are inserted. If there's one statement about what to eat that approaches absolute truth, it's this: *somebody must be wrong or misinformed; otherwise, the food conundrums and contradictions wouldn't be so pervasive.*

We suggest that food contradictions and diet battles seem to propagate via three overarching ideas: 1) believing nutrition is an emergency; 2) macroconfusion, resulting from grouping foods by biochemical structures that aren't metabolically similar; and 3) chronic overnutrition driven by social eating pressures and fear of deficiency. These three concepts have likely induced an insidious creep to a chronically fed state from birth to death in all populations as access to food increases.

How can we reconcile the social drive toward chronic overnutrition with a nearly unanimous outcome of longevity research on diet intervention concluding the benefits result from antithesis: dietary restriction without malnutrition? What are the important lessons in nutrition now that year-round access to food is no longer economically or environmentally scarce? Is it time for us to move past the fear of deficiency given the overwhelming evidence that less is more?

CHAPTER 3

HEALTHSPAN HABITS

NUTRITION IS NOT AN EMERGENCY

Diet recently surpassed smoking as the number one cause of early death and disability in the U.S.[1] In 2019, this expanded to the global level.[2] For the first time in human history, we are seeing a global shift toward a double burden of malnutrition, when both under- and overnutrition exist simultaneously within the same society.[3] In the not-so-distant past, people struggled to attain enough food to survive. Scarcity was at the center of the economy, and not having enough was a real threat to physiological security. Diseases caused by deficiency, such as rickets, beriberi, and goiters, were not uncommon, and that is why we ended up with commercial foods such as iodine-enriched salt, vitamin D–fortified milk, and B vitamin–enriched bread. Despite the complete flip toward more ubiquitous access to calories, healthcare education remains predicated upon the avoidance of deficiency.

We continue to spend most of our time worried about getting enough nutrition, while most of the world is suffering from too much. Nutrition is not an emergency. For many years, we defended a plant-based diet in terms of its adequacy in nutrition. Yet, when we examine the data on healthspan and longevity, a perhaps surprising hypothesis begins to surface. What if the myriad health advantages of a plant-based diet are due to the fact that it's naturally restricted in certain nutrients? Eating this way seems to activate many of the same longevity pathways associated with dietary restriction, while providing adequate nutrition for all.[4][5][6]

Macroconfusion

All energy in food comes from some combination of proteins, carbohydrates, and fats. Alcohol also provides calories (7 per gram), but these calories are not considered essential in the diet. Macronutrient ratios form the basis of hotly contested debates, with most centered on the nonprotein energy balance (e.g., low/high carb versus low/high fat). We believe this is one of the predominant reasons for almost ubiquitous confusion about what to eat. It seems to create confusion about food with the layperson, media, researchers, and healthcare providers. There are plenty of examples supporting healthful benefits on all sides of the macronutrient ratio spectrum, from the Mediterranean diet, which might be higher in certain fats, to a traditional Okinawan diet, which is low in fat. This apparent contradiction suggests that the actual quality of food consumed may matter more than the purely macronutrient ratio. The food-health connection is complex, and macronutrients don't have enough specificity to address the wide-ranging

> "What if the myriad health advantages of a plant-based diet are due to the fact that it's naturally restricted in certain nutrients?"

issues. Often, this conflict results in confusion that pushes people to frustration and apathy. We call this *macroconfusion*. We want to yank our plate conversation out of biochemistry and return it to discussing food.

We know the words "protein," "carbohydrate," and "fat" likely evoke images of food in your mind. These categories of food have existed since first introduced by William Prout in 1834.[7] At that time, science was undergoing a revolution to understand the metabolic underpinning of life. By the close of the nineteenth century, these component fuels became not only food groupings, but more importantly, units of economic equivalency. Food took on a new meaning, and what we eat became inextricably intertwined with a more nuanced, technical description. One concept that's grown out of control is how Liebig's protein-plus-fuel categorization of food has completely permeated the food supply chain. Let's take a closer look at the P-word, C-word, and F-word and how these biochemical food obscenities have created division and may contribute to us knowing more and understanding less about food.

Protein

Proteins are the building blocks of life. They form the basis for every structure and function in all living organisms, enzymes, fibers, hormones, antibodies, etc. Here's a fun fact that will help you step away from macroconfusion: protein isn't a food group. An egg isn't a protein. Eggs contain protein, but so do potatoes, legumes, bananas, and all living organisms. It's even more nuanced because every living cell, potato and chicken alike, contains thousands of proteins (plural). The protein label is analogous to calling something a metal, which isn't adequate to capture the important material variations in iron, aluminum, or gold. When considered from an application perspective, these metals each have different properties. Likewise, the general category of "protein" isn't descriptive enough in a dietary sense to say much about health. We need to know more.

Generally speaking, there are 20 amino acids that act much like the 26 letters of the alphabet. When one eats and digests plant or animal protein, it's broken down into the individual constituent amino acids (letters) and our cells create the words, sentences, and paragraphs of our genetic book of life. No animal makes all 20 amino acids. It's a little like protein Jeopardy and we must "buy a vowel,"— the essential amino acids—through diet to complete the protein words. The DNA of all organisms is the blueprint for the tens of thousands of different proteins that make up all living cells. Animals, unlike plants, must acquire some of the amino acid building blocks, the essential amino acids, through diet. The amino acids are used as starting material and transformed through cellular processes into the myriad proteins required for all of our various structures and physiological functions. We actually don't have a need for dietary protein in a strict biological sense. Rather, we need a nitrogen source to synthesize the non-essential amino acids and a dietary source of essential amino acids—a subset of amino acids we can't make ourselves.

Every whole plant food, from grapes to beans, contains *all amino acids*. Plants can't eat, which means they must synthesize all 20 amino acids. And while individual amino acid *concentrations* vary from plant to plant or from plant to animal, they are all there. This is made obvious when one considers that the 10 largest, most muscular land mammals (five species of rhinoceroses, two species of elephants, a hippopotamus, a giraffe, and a gaur), eat only plant-sourced food and have no problem getting sufficient protein and essential amino acids. Animals, including humans, can eat plants, rupture the cell walls through mastication, digest these plant proteins through proteolytic enzymes, and absorb amino acids for ribosomal protein synthesis. The process is identical whether the protein originated from an animal or a plant cell. Despite the dietary need for essential amino acids, the 10 to 25,000 different proteins are synthesized in cellular ribosomes. Proteins are synthesized in our cells and don't originate in diet.

Certain essential amino acids—for example, those amino acids that longevity and healthspan research suggest should be limited or restricted, such as methionine, leucine, and lysine—are naturally limited in plant-sourced food. This is likely a component of the health successes seen in the mostly plant-based Mediterranean and Okinawan diets. Here is the take-home message for everyone about protein: we eat the plant or we eat the animal that ate the plant, but the necessary dietary essential amino acids originated in the plant or bacteria.

Carbohydrate

Cotton, paper, wood, fructose, and glucose are all *carbohydrates*. While it's common to use the "carbs" label for whole foods such as potatoes, legumes, and rice, it's probably not a very accurate way to categorize these foods. Would anyone question whether glucose and wood were metabolically similar in a meal? Probably not, and yet, the cellulose of wood is a long chain of glucose. Termites have the enzyme to break down cellulose to glucose, and humans don't. While carbohydrates share chemical similarity, they are not necessarily *isometabolic*, or metabolically equivalent.

A whole potato isn't isometabolic with highly processed junk food, such as potato chips or French fries. This has lead to some poor national food policy positions and consumer guidelines. In Jennifer Woolfe's scholarly work *The Potato in the*

"We eat the plant or we eat the animal that ate the plant, but the necessary dietary essential amino acids originated in the plant or bacteria."

BAKED POTATO	90% LEAN BEEF

Nutrition Facts
Serving Size 100 grams

Amount Per Serving

Calories 93	Calories from Fat 1
	% Daily Value*
Total Fat 0g	0%
Saturated Fat 0g	0%
Trans Fat	
Cholesterol 0mg	0%
Sodium 10mg	0%
Total Carbohydrate 21g	7%
Dietary Fiber 2g	9%
Sugars 1g	
Protein 3g	

Vitamin A	0%	•	Vitamin C	16%
Calcium	1%	•	Iron	6%

*Percent Daily Values are based on a 2,000 calorie diet. Your daily values may be higher or lower depending on your calorie needs.

109
Amino Acid Score

Nutrition Facts
Serving Size 100 grams

Amount Per Serving

Calories 230	Calories from Fat 109
	% Daily Value*
Total Fat 12g	19%
Saturated Fat 5g	24%
Trans Fat 1g	
Cholesterol 89mg	30%
Sodium 87mg	4%
Total Carbohydrate 0g	0%
Dietary Fiber 0g	0%
Sugars 0g	
Protein 28g	

Vitamin A	0%	•	Vitamin C	0%
Calcium	2%	•	Iron	17%

*Percent Daily Values are based on a 2,000 calorie diet. Your daily values may be higher or lower depending on your calorie needs.

79
Amino Acid Score

Equal weight potato versus beef comparison of amino acid profile to that recommended by the Institute of Medicine's Food and Nutrition Board. (source: USDA//Self Nutrition Data)

daily requirement of vitamin K, riboflavin, pantothenic acid, zinc, and calcium. Using data from the USDA nutrient database to back this up, a baked potato actually has a better amino acid score than 90-percent lean beef. (Here, a score of 100 or more refers to nutritionally ideal but not necessarily ideal for healthspan.) In *Plant-Based Nutrition,* Second Edition,[9] we discuss in more detail simple versus complex carbohydrates and concepts such as glycemic index, but you're better off to drop all of these labels and move toward using whole-food descriptions. It's better to use "carrot" and avoid using "low-glycemic, complex carbohydrate." What should be clear, with nearly unlimited access to food and with the prevalence of chronic overnutrition, is that calling a potato a "carb" is simply unhealthful.[10] If the word "carbohydrate" didn't exist, how else could we group disparate substances like cotton, paper, beans, potatoes, doughnuts, and rice together? Would anyone really place a wonderful lentil stew in the same category as the average fortified, sugar-laden, breakfast cereal? Of course not, and yet there are plenty of double-blind, randomized, controlled crossover "gold standard" diet trials juggling macronutrient ratios that unintentionally do just that. "Compared to what?" is the question not asked often enough. By

Human Diet, she points out that contrary to the popular notion that potatoes are rich sources of energy and poor sources of protein, vitamins, and minerals, evidence is clear that unless fried, potatoes contain high-quality protein and are rich in micronutrients.[8] If one eats enough potato to meet a daily 2,000-calorie requirement, a potato can become a sole source of dietary protein, vitamin C, niacin, vitamin B6, folate, iron, magnesium, phosphorous, potassium, copper, and manganese. In addition, it provides more than half of the organizing food in these isoenergetic groups, we've created an unimaginable mess and fueled endless, unproductive carb versus fat debates.

Fats

Like we've seen with the amino acids of proteins and the various starches, sugars, and fibers of carbohydrates, not all lipids are isometabolic despite being isocaloric. Two energetically identical lipid molecules may have profoundly different health impacts.

The terms "saturated" and "unsaturated" refer to the chemical structure of the fat molecular chains. When hydrogens are removed from a saturated fat, the adjacent carbon atoms form double bonds, each replacing the bond it previously shared with a removed hydrogen with another carbon. We call this hydrogen removal "unsaturation" because hydrogen no longer "saturates" every available location. This means the remaining hydrogens attached to these carbons can either end up on the same side (cis) or on opposite sides (trans), and this greatly impacts the chemistry of the molecules. Generally speaking, saturated fats are found primarily in animal products. The molecular chains are very linear. Like straight hair, they pack densely and become solid at higher temperatures. On the other hand, plant fats tend to be unsaturated, which creates a kink at the naturally occurring cis double bond. The kink interferes with packing, and these fats tend to remain liquid at lower temperatures.

For example, consider placing olive oil and an animal fat in the refrigerator. Olive oil, an unsaturated fat often found in salad dressings, doesn't solidify, whereas the saturated fat of pork, beef, or chicken stock will form a solidified layer on top. Likewise, coconut oil is higher in saturated fat than olive oil and solidifies at room temperatures. This confirms that even plant-based oils exhibit identical liquid versus solid, unsaturated versus saturated fat properties.

Recognizing the potential health benefits of limiting saturated fats and the lower cost of plant oils, hydrogenation was introduced by food companies to make unsaturated plant fats spread and cook like animal-sourced saturated fats people were accustomed to using. Saturated and unsaturated fats behave differently at room temperature, allowing us to spread butter (saturated) on the bread or dip the bread into liquid olive oil (unsaturated). This ushered in partial hydrogenation—making plant oils spread like butter—but this process created a new health issue: trans fatty acids. Today, everyone seems to agree about the health issues associated with trans fats, and they were banned in 2015 by the FDA.[11] Our recommendation is that all fats be primarily sourced from whole-plant foods, not oils or butters, and these will be primarily monounsaturated and polyunsaturated fatty acids.

THE FOOD TRIANGLE: A NEW MODEL FOR YOUR PLATE

In spite of their utility in biochemistry, the macronutrient labeling scheme is more a tool of marketing and food propaganda than of health. In 2014, Ray and his collaborators at Harvard and the National Institute of Health (NIH) introduced the *Food Triangle*, a new paradigm to conceptualize food that captures the energy density component as well as the contribution to healthspan and longevity.[12] They expanded this concept in 2017 with their paper on *oxidative priority*—to address more subtle metabolic underpinnings or perceived macronutrient energy contradictions as they relate to obesity.[13] Together, we integrated this concept into a general

plant-based guide for healthcare professionals to implement diet as a primary intervention for chronic disease.[14] Following the Food Triangle will take most of the guesswork out of making food decisions.

The Food Triangle is based entirely on whole foods. It doesn't address food adulterants such as sugars, salt, oils, and flours, which we will expound upon in Chapter 4. At the apex, leafy greens, cruciferous vegetables, stems (e.g., asparagus and celery), bulbs (e.g., garlic and onions), and mushrooms are foods that become the nutritional foundation of

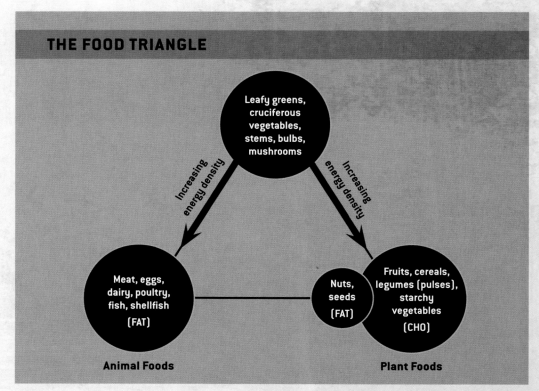

THE FOOD TRIANGLE

Leafy greens, cruciferous vegetables, stems, bulbs, mushrooms

Increasing energy density

Increasing energy density

Meat, eggs, dairy, poultry, fish, shellfish (FAT)

Nuts, seeds (FAT)

Fruits, cereals, legumes (pulses), starchy vegetables (CHO)

Animal Foods

Plant Foods

The Food Triangle is a simple way to organize foods while eliminating the shortcomings of the protein, carbohydrate, and fat labeling. At a glance, one can recognize that foods at the top and right are high in fiber and phytonutrients, lower in saturated fats, and restricted (not deficient) in certain amino acids. Carbohydrate (CHO), Fat (FAT)

daily meals, rather than the more energy-dense alternatives at the bottom. They provide a rich source of phytonutrients and can be eaten in nearly unlimited quantities.

Down one side of the Food Triangle, we see increasing calorie content and nutrition from animal-sourced food; down the other side, we see plant-sourced food. As it turns out, both left- and right-side eating share certain short-term benefits when compared to bottom feeding, and this may bias people toward decisions that give immediate improvement with long-term detriment.

Left-Side Eating

The Atkins, paleo, and keto diets mostly consist of foods from the left side of the Food Triangle. Eating this way can be used to control weight, as it tends to limit the starchy foods on the right side. Sometimes, people on these diets further limit animal-sourced foods such as dairy or red meat, and others limit or eliminate plant food entirely. Eating toward the left and eliminating starchy vegetables, grains, and fruits reduces the diet's available caloric content, and this is one of the main reasons for its success. When one decreases from chronically overnourished to proper levels of nourishment, we *should* see positive health benefits. However, moving in a beneficial direction doesn't automatically imply optimal nutrition.

Left-side eating focuses on foods that are high in saturated fat, heme iron, essential amino acids, N-glycolylneuraminic acid (Neu5Gc), carnitine, and chemical contaminants that are formed when flesh is cooked, such as polycyclic aromatic hydrocarbons, heterocyclic amines, and advanced glycation end products. There is evidence that some of these (e.g., higher dietary amino acid levels) may favor reproductive prime, athletic performance, or evolutionary success yet disfavor longevity and healthspan. We may be biased in a world that holds competitive athletes in nearly unquestionable high esteem, representing the pinnacle of human health, but it may be an evolutionary trade-off without significant long-term benefits.[15][16] It's hard to study eating patterns over the 80 to 100 years of human life, but studies of many other organisms point consistently to "less is more."

Bottom Feeding

A Western diet, which is becoming increasingly common worldwide, tends to be focused more on the bottom of the Food Triangle. In fact, if one thinks of most cultural food recipes, they tend to be constructed from the bottom of the Food Triangle: steak and potatoes, fish and chips, burgers and fries, curry and rice, meat sauce and pasta, and a host of soups and stews. These are often combined with excess sugars, salt, oils, and flours, which further enhance excessive energy intake and poor-health food choices. Bottom feeding makes for the most energy-dense meals, and obesity and chronic overnourishment is its likely unintended consequence.

Right-Side Eating

The right side of the Food Triangle emphasizes energy from plant-sourced, whole-food starches and sugars found in fruits, cereals, legumes, and starchy vegetables. There are some exceptions containing more fat such as nuts, seeds, avocados, and coconuts. Nuts and seeds are an excellent source of phytonutrients and the required 1 to 3 percent of the essential fatty acids required in the diet. Similar to left-side eating, right-side eating limits the overall energy value of the diet. Like left-side eating and bottom feeding, eating exclusively plant-sourced food can be subject to excess food adulteration with sugars, salt, oils, and flours.

We've seen the negative impacts of chronic overnutrition in bottom feeding, and most won't question the added burden of highly processed and adulterated food. Likewise, there's been a surge in the last decade of plant-sourced junk foods such as burgers, hot dogs,

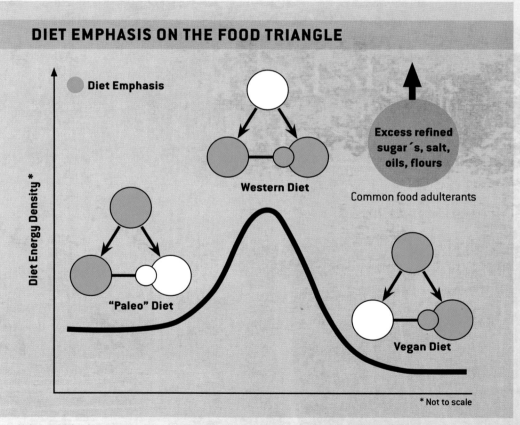

DIET EMPHASIS ON THE FOOD TRIANGLE

Diet Emphasis

Diet Energy Density *

Western Diet

Excess refined sugar´s, salt, oils, flours

Common food adulterants

"Paleo" Diet

Vegan Diet

* Not to scale

Using the left-, right-, and bottom-feeding paradigms, relative diet scheme calorie restriction and excess is easily visualized. Adding excess refined food adulterants can further tip the scale toward overnutrition.

dairy-free processed cheese, cakes, cookies, and so on, along with decadent, hyperpalatable, exclusively plant-sourced restaurants. Over that same decade, Julieanna has seen a rise in clients eating a plant-based diet in her dietetics counseling practice who present with the same issues (e.g., high blood pressure, diabetes, and high lipid panels), previously seen only in clients eating an omnivorous diet.

Oxidative Priority

Before leaving the Food Triangle, we'd like to touch upon the implications of one more concept that may impact how you eat, particularly when battling weight creep. One reason bottom feeding is so economically frugal is a result of how our body prioritizes ingested calories. We will return the discussion to the macronutrients, but this time, we don't want you to think of them as food groups, rather, as simply energy components of food. You'll need a couple of assumptions to begin this discussion. First, our bodies don't generally convert excess calories, other than ingested fat, into adipose fat stores. Transforming dietary protein (amino acids), alcohol, carbohydrate, or their metabolites into fat is called *de novo lipogenesis,* and it's an insignificant contribution to your body's fat stores.[17] Secondly, our bodies have limited storage capacity for excess alcohol (none), protein (amino acids; 380–420 kcal), and carbohydrate (about 500–2,000 kcal). Now let's compare this to dietary fat storage capacity.

It's certainly not uncommon for people today to be 50 to 100 pounds overweight, and humans have reached 600 to 800 pounds or more. Let's stop to put that in caloric perspective. If we use human fat tissue as the calorie standard, every 100 pounds is 350,000 calories or nearly 1,000 calories a day over a year. In the absence of creating fat from surplus energy, we have extremely limited potential to store excessive alcohol, amino acids, and starches or sugars. Equally important is that the body must have mechanisms to prevent us from storing all the extra energy we eat over weeks and months. Consider that gaining 50 pounds over 20 years—certainly a reasonable pathway to an obese status for most of us—is the dietary equivalent of an extra 168 calories *per week*. Who guesses their caloric content in an entire week to within ¾ cup of brown rice, 3½ ounces of salmon, or 1½ glasses of wine? Likely no one counts calories to this level; this is the calorie equivalent of 16 peanut M&Ms or 56 plain M&Ms.

How does oxidative priority account for this accumulation of fat? The rise and fall is a general pattern that lasts about 4 to 6 hours (sometimes longer). The process begins with blood levels of nutrients at a normal level pre-meal. A mixed-nutrient meal is consumed. Then 4 to 6 hours later, the blood nutrient concentration has returned to pre-meal levels. Where did the meal go? Let's assume you burned through 80 to 100 calories per hour in those 4 to 6 hours. Our meals are often larger than 600

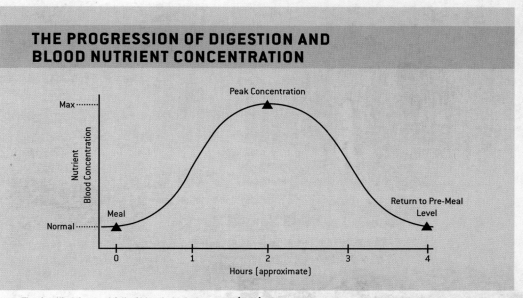

THE PROGRESSION OF DIGESTION AND BLOOD NUTRIENT CONCENTRATION

The familiar rise and fall of blood alcohol content (BAC) after drinking also occurs with glucose, amino acids, and lipids after eating. The body's attempt to bring these post-meal rises back to normal—homeostasis combined with limited storage capacity for each energy source—drives oxidative priority.

calories, perhaps 3,000 calories on a night out at a restaurant or Thanksgiving holiday meal. And yet when one measures circulating blood nutrient concentration hours after the meal, they've returned to pre-meal levels.

Oxidative priority hypothesizes that calories consumed are prioritized to metabolize in the reverse order of their storage capacity. Alcohol can't be stored and is metabolized with the highest priority, whereas fat has nearly unlimited storage capacity relative to any one meal and is the lowest priority. Amino acids and glucose share metabolic pathways, and both have limited storage. If we don't store these higher priority calories, where did they go? It appears that your body temporarily increases its total energy

output and shifts priority to the calories that can't be stored. You've probably experienced overheating in bed following an unusually large meal or too much alcohol. Perhaps you've noticed how late-night meals disrupt sleep. We produce waste heat with most of the food swallowed. This is true of your car as well; most of the fuel energy in the tank is used to heat the engine, exhaust, and brakes. Our bodies seem to have cleverly adapted to hanging onto fat for later, but later never comes. As summarized in our oxidative priority paper,

...one can translate these results to what occurs when an individual consumes a wine, cheese, and cracker hors d'oeuvre. The post-hors d'oeuvre rise in alcohol and glucose concentrations actually suppresses fat oxidation and promotes storage of the dietary fat from the meal. As such, one can easily understand how body fat increases over time; the homeostatic drive to normalize postprandial rises in blood nutrient levels offers a novel conceptual framework that predicts fat accumulation.

Now take a look at bottom feeding on the Food Triangle again. Not only is bottom feeding higher in overall calories, but it's also a very efficient way to *maximize* fat storage. The low-fat crowd blames the fat, and the low-carb crowd blames the carbohydrate. They are both correct, but not for the reasons offered. Sugar isn't converted to fat (*de novo lipogenesis*) in any appreciable level and fat swallowed isn't instantly shuffled to your love handles.[18] [19] [20] [21] [22] [23] [24] The process is far more complicated and insidious, and fat accumulation isn't the only health metric. We also must address the other nutritional elements—both beneficial and detrimental—that should be selectively increased or diminished in diet.

The Food Triangle is a simple mnemonic to do a quick check on meals and drop the former protein, carbohydrate, and fat labels that are the source of macroconfusion. We simply say, "Keep eating right." The bulk of your meals should come from the top and bottom right of the Food Triangle to meet

> **"The bulk of your meals should come from the top of the Food Triangle."**

calorie needs. To further guide you, we created two additional Food Triangle variations that are targeted at those who have eliminated some or all animal products from their diet due to health or ideological consideration.

The same guidelines for left-side eating, right-side eating, and bottom feeding apply to those following a vegetarian or vegan diet. In particular, vegetarians are probably the most exposed to bottom feeding in a deleterious manner. The dairy-starch combination is likely a large part of the Western diet dilemma, and this cheese-and-pasta style of eating should not be overlooked. For those who have eliminated all animal products, nuts, seeds, avocado, coconut, and oils are the primary fat sources, and of course, flours and added sugars are the other food elements of caution. These ingredients aren't an acute detriment, but they can unintentionally slip into the diet in excessive amounts, increasing food palatability, and driving plant-sourced overnutrition.

Our message isn't to condemn these outright or ban them from the plate. We believe that these few adulterants are easy to recognize and restrict. In the recipes, we've limited these ingredients, but we expect some may protest our deviation from complete abstinence. We've also not taken the moderation approach; some recipes are nearly perfect in composition, others are excellent, and still others are good. Compared to the standard Western diet, all the recipes in this book are a huge improvement.

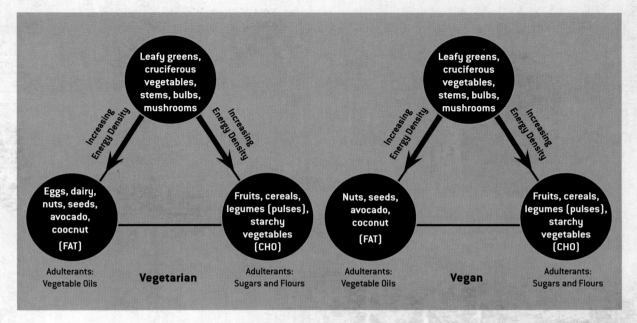

Vegetarians and vegans who limit most or all animal-sourced food should consider using an alternative Food Triangle to easily segregate food. The rise in these options over the last couple of decades has introduced more refined food adulterants into the meals along with an associated rise in health-related issues. Carbohydrate (CHO), Fat (FAT)

We hope this makes it easier to understand why the fruitarians and the carnivores can't seem to agree. It's an explanation similar to the "yanny and laurel" audio illusion or the "blue and gold dress" visual illusion; search online if you haven't seen these. Using the original Food Triangle or one specifically for animal-free menus will help you visualize how the calories inch in over time without becoming an anti-nut, -oil, or -sugar avenger. We sincerely hope you'll permanently drop the protein, carbohydrate, and fat labels causing macroconfusion, and keep eating right on the Food Triangle. There are many nuanced elements beyond the elimination of macronutrient food groupings. Next,

we'll explore the fantastic world of plant-sourced vitamins, minerals, fiber, and phytonutrients.

NOTABLE NUTRIENTS

Before we discuss the few nutrients that may be limited by sticking to the right side of the Food Triangle, let's explore the extraordinary offerings that are unique to plant foods: fiber and phytonutrients.

Dietary Fiber

Dietary fiber is a broad category of long chains of complex carbohydrates— "unavailable carbohydrate," as it was first described[25] —that are resistant to digestion. Despite the fact that fiber provides copious health advantages, consumption around the globe is less than half of what is recommended.[26] There is ample evidence that this fiber gap is contributing to a disappearing microbiome, which is implicated in the expanding prevalence of chronic disease.[27]

We host about 38 trillion microbial cells.[28] A large percentage of these microbial cells live in our gastrointestinal tract, and these diverse communities—collectively known as the microbiome—play a key role in human health via powerful metabolic, immunologic, and protective functions.[29] With the ever-expanding understanding of this symbiotic relationship, dietary fiber is more and more consequential in dictating our general health and disease-fighting capabilities. Because fiber comes exclusively from plant foods, emphasizing right-side triangle eating offers opportunities to meet recommended intakes and benefit from these compounds.

There are multiple classifications of dietary fiber that encompass some of the specific roles each plays in our bodies, mostly through bulking, viscosity, and fermentation.[30] Broadly speaking, fibers are categorized as soluble or insoluble, though this definition is limiting because of the diverse physiological and physicochemical properties of these various compounds.

Here are some examples of different types of dietary fibers, their benefits, and their sources:

Insoluble fibers include mainly celluloses, hemicelluloses, and lignins, which are found in all whole-plant foods; they are associated with improved digestion and bowel health, removal of metabolic waste from the body, and enhanced satiety.
Prebiotics are defined as substrates that are selectively utilized by host microorganisms conferring health benefits.[31] While "all prebiotics are fiber, not all fiber is prebiotic." The fermentation of these fibers results in the production of short-chain fatty acids (SCFA), which reduce pathogenic bacteria and enhance healthful bacteria in the gut.[32] [33]
Soluble fibers either dissolve or swell to form a gel with water and include:

- *Beta glucans*, which act as prebiotics and may offer antitumor, immune-enhancing, bone-healing, anti-diabetic, and cholesterol- and blood pressure-lowering benefits, are found in cereals (mainly barley and oats) and mushrooms.[34]

- *Pectins* also act as prebiotics and have been associated with enhancing excretion of toxic metals and improving cholesterol profiles and blood glucose levels. They can be found in all plants, especially in citrus fruits and apples, and they are attractive for their gel-forming capability, perfect for jams and jellies.[35] [36]

"Fiber is likely one of the most significant factors for the healthspan-promoting effects of a diet emphasizing whole plant foods."

- *Gums and mucilages*, found in sea vegetables and plant seeds, may serve as prebiotics and support digestive function and health; they are used to thicken, emulsify, stabilize, and texturize in the food industry.[37] [38]

- *Resistant starches* are fermentable, exerting prebiotic effects, potentially reducing colorectal cancer risk, and aiding in the management of diabetes and weight. They are found primarily in legumes as well as unripened bananas, cooked and cooled potatoes, and cereal grains.[39]

- *Inulin-type fructans* also employ prebiotic effects and are found in many foods including leeks, asparagus, onions, wheat, garlic, chicory, oats, soybeans, and Jerusalem artichokes.[40]

Beyond this list, there is an expanding database of types of dietary fibers, and their myriad advantages continue to emerge, particularly with regard to their intricate interconnection to the gut microbiome.

En masse, as a nutrient group, dietary fiber can reduce the risk for type 2 diabetes and cardiovascular disease, improve and protect gastrointestinal health, help reduce excess sex hormones and toxins (such as heavy metals), and enhance satiation and satiety. Fiber is likely one of the most significant factors for the healthspan-promoting effects of a diet emphasizing whole-plant foods.

Phytonutrients

Phytonutrients are the other enormously critical category of nutrients that provide a plethora of plant-powered benefits. Since plants cannot run or hide, they produce compounds in order to protect themselves from pathogens, predators, injury, weather, drought, and other stressors to which they are exposed. They also contain compounds that are responsible for their color, flavor, aroma, and texture. Collectively, these chemicals are referred to as phytochemicals (*phyto* is Greek for "plant") or phytonutrients because many of these exert powerful positive effects on the humans who consume them.

While about 4,000 different compounds have been identified thus far, hundreds have been studied and, as with dietary fiber, new and exciting data continue to emerge. Defined as nonnutritive, naturally occurring biochemicals, phytonutrients can be divided and subdivided into many different categories based on their chemical structure and function. Five of the most common categories include carotenoids, flavonoids, curcumin, organosulfur compounds, and phytosterols.[41]

Carotenoids: of the 750 fat-soluble carotenoids found in nature, about 50 contain provitamin activity, and only three are considered significant precursors for vitamin A in humans, which is needed for development, growth, immune function, and vision. Of the 40 carotenoids present in the human diet, 90 percent are represented by beta-carotene, alpha-carotene, lycopene, lutein, and cryptoxanthin. Carotenoids are responsible for the red, orange, and yellow colors in foods (e.g., tomatoes and sweet potatoes). They are also present in dark green leafy vegetables (e.g., spinach and broccoli), but the colors are masked by the chlorophyll pigment. Besides being a source of provitamin A, carotenoids also act as powerful antioxidants, protect the skin and eyes, and offer cardioprotective, anti-inflammatory, antimutagenic, and anticarcinogenic activities.[42 43]

Flavonoids encompass the largest group of antioxidants and can be subdivided into flavones, flavonols, flavanones, flavanonols, flavanols or catechins, anthocyanins, and chalcones.[44] Considered indispensable in many nutraceutical, pharmaceutical, medicinal, and cosmetic applications, this large family of over 5,000 compounds can be found ubiquitously in plants. Flavonoids offer sirtuin-activating, antioxidative, anti-inflammatory, antimicrobial, antimutagenic, and anticarcinogenic properties and a capacity to modulate key cellular enzyme function. The most concentrated sources of flavonoids are fruits (particularly citrus fruits), vegetables, tea, red wine, and legumes.

Also included in this category are isoflavone, which are found in soyfoods and other legumes and associated with an essential role in the reduction of carcinogenesis (especially hormone-dependent cancer) and diabetes, and in protecting bones and the cardiovascular and central nervous systems.[45]

Isoflavonoids are one of the nutrient groups highlighted in the Okinawan diet, particularly from soyfoods. Soy's isoflavones are also associated with hormetic properties that can activate cell-signaling pathways that are strongly associated with healthy aging and longevity.[46 47 48]

Curcumin, another phytonutrient ascribed to traditional Okinawa's exceptional diet, is the fat-soluble polyphenol responsible for the yellow color of turmeric, a root derived from the ginger family that contains potent medicinal properties. Like soy's isoflavones, curcumin also affects hormesis, which supports healthspan and aids in the management of oxidative and inflammatory conditions, metabolic syndrome, arthritis, anxiety, and hyperlipidemia.[49]

Organosulfur compounds are a broad category that happen to encompass two extraordinarily healthful phytonutrients—allicin and sulforaphane. Garlic contains allicin, an active enzyme that offers antimicrobial, antihypertensive, antithrombotic, and anticancer benefits. To derive optimal benefits, eat it raw and also crush or cut the garlic and wait 10 minutes before consuming it so the enzyme alliinase can metabolize alliin to allicin.[50 51] Glucosinolates—sulfur-containing compounds found in cruciferous vegetables, especially broccoli, cabbage, cauliflower, and kale—are converted into biologically active isothiocyanates, including sulforaphane, when released by chopping or chewing via the myrosinase enzyme. Sulforaphane

> **"... set a daily goal to 'eat the rainbow.'"**

provides potent chemopreventive, detoxifying, neuroprotective, anti-inflammatory, anticarcinogenic, antioxidant, and broad spectrum antimicrobial properties.[52][53] Interestingly, the myrosinase enzyme is deactivated when cooked, which lowers the bioavailability of sulforaphane. Adding mustard (ground from seeds or powdered) to cruciferous vegetables after they have been cooked provides ample myrosinase to ensure adequate conversion to these active compounds.[54][55]

Phytosterols, as the name implies, are plant compounds similar in structure to cholesterol. High intakes of phytosterols can lower serum total and low-density lipoprotein-cholesterol concentrations in humans. Along with soy, almonds, and viscous fibers (e.g., oats, barley, okra, and eggplant), phytosterols in the Portfolio diet were able to reduce cholesterol at the same level as statins.[56][57][58] They have also been associated with sirtuin-activating, anticancer, and anti-inflammatory effects and can be found in all plant foods, but concentrations are particularly high in legumes, nuts, seeds, and cereals.[59]

All plants contain a variety of different compounds that work synergistically in our bodies to produce widespread advantages, including their sirtuin-activating, antioxidant, anti-inflammatory, anticancer, anti-obesity, immunostimulating, detoxifying, antiatherogenic, chemopreventive, antiosteoporotic, and antimicrobial activities.[60][61] Despite efforts, isolating and concentrating these nutrients into supplements does not always have the same effect as when consumed intact from the food.

Foods that contain phytonutrients are—of course—plant foods, but sources that tend to contain the highest levels include cruciferous vegetables; leafy green vegetables; dark orange and red fruits and vegetables, such as berries, cherries, plums, and tomatoes; soyfoods; spices such as turmeric; and tea. To summarize the intended practical advice from the extensive literature review of this broad area of study, simply set a daily goal to "eat the rainbow."

With this impressive catalogue of benefits bestowed upon us when we consume plant foods—particularly from their fibers and phytonutrients, but also from what we are avoiding by eschewing animal products (e.g., excessive amino acids, saturated fat, and heme iron)—the long-term, healthspan-enhancing impact seems evident.

ESSENTIAL NUTRIENTS

With all of that goodness in mind, there is a short list of nutrients to be mindful of when eating on the right side of the Food Triangle: vitamins B12, D, and K2; iodine; zinc; and the long-chain omega-3 fatty acids, eicosapentaenoic acid (EPA), and docosahexaenoic acid (DHA).

Vitamin B12

One of the key nutrients that needs to be addressed is cobalamin, commonly referred to as vitamin B12. This water-soluble vitamin will eventually fall short for people eating on the right side of the triangle, as well as anyone over the age of 60 (regardless of diet), those with certain gastrointestinal absorption issues (e.g., celiac disease and Crohn's disease), and those who take certain medications (e.g., proton pump inhibitors and metformin).[62]

Vitamin B12 is produced by microorganisms, bacteria, fungi, and algae but not by animals or plants. It is found in animal products because after ingesting these microorganisms along with their food, animals concentrate B12 in their flesh, organs, and byproducts (e.g., eggs and dairy). Further, ruminant animals (such as cows, sheep, and goats) have bacteria in their rumen that produce vitamin B12. We need this nutrient for neurological function, the creation of DNA, and red blood cell production, as well as participation in myriad metabolic reactions.

Although you can find vitamin B12 in fortified foods, such as plant milks, cereals, and nutritional yeast, these are mostly inadequate and unreliable sources. The risk for serious health complications due to a deficiency is too high to not take seriously; these health risks include potentially irreversible neurological disorders, gastrointestinal problems, and megaloblastic anemia. Despite claims that certain plant foods (fermented foods, spirulina, chlorella, certain mushrooms,

and sea vegetables) can provide B12, the vitamin is not usually biologically active. These inactive compounds act as analogues, which makes them able to attach to B12 receptors and thereby may prevent absorption of the functional form.[63]

Interestingly, the body is able to store B12 for at least three to five years. To further complicate this, signs and symptoms for deficiency are either not noticeable or are subtle, and there can be a 5- to 10-year delay from the onset of deficiency to the manifestation of symptoms.[64] If B12 is not being consumed at adequate levels or if there are absorption problems, deficiency will eventually ensue. Because blood tests for B12 levels can be skewed by other variables, irreversible damage may occur before a deficiency is detected.

Recommended dietary allowances (RDAs) for vitamin B12 across the lifespan vary from 0.4 micrograms for infants to 2.8 micrograms for lactating women. For nonpregnant adults aged 14 and above, the RDA is 2.4 micrograms per day. To ensure this is absorbed (in a healthy individual, barring any possible inhibitors), higher doses are recommended.

The bottom line is that it seems the best way for adults to maximize absorption and maintain optimal blood levels is to supplement with one of these dosing regimens of vitamin B12: 50 micrograms twice a day, 150 micrograms once a day, or 2,500 micrograms once a week. There are different forms of cobalamin that you can find in supplement form, including cyanocobalamin and methylcobalamin. Cyanocobalamin appears to be the most stable, economical, and safe form, which is why it is most commonly used in research and, therefore, the form we recommend.[65]

High doses of B12 are safe, and a tolerable upper limit has not been established. It is best to undergo testing of serum cobalamin and methylmalonic acid, as this latter test is considered the most sensitive test for deficiency. Modify your dose as necessary, as per your physician's guidance.[66]

Vitamin D

Calciferol, commonly known as vitamin D or the "sunshine vitamin," is unique. It is a prohormone produced in the skin upon exposure to UVB rays from the sun. Vitamin D deficiency is now considered a global epidemic.[67] [68] [69] Many factors, including excessive sunscreen use, indoor lifestyles, smog, and latitude, among others, contribute to many people falling short on this crucial nutrient. Deficiency is implicated in a wide range of issues, such as osteoporosis, cardiovascular disease, autoimmune disease, and much more.

Clearly, this is a vitamin to pay attention to. Standard protocol is to regularly check levels of serum 25-hydroxyvitamin D. According to the National Institutes of Health, serum levels of at least 20 ng/mL (50 nmol/L) meet the needs of 97.5 percent of the population and are considered adequate for bone health and overall health in healthy individuals.[70] Interestingly, there is evidence to justify higher optimal levels of 30 ng/mL (75 nmol/L) or more for chronic disease prevention.[71] [72]

Sun therapy may help meet at least some of your vitamin D requirement. You should get 5 to 30 minutes of sun exposure at peak hours (usually 10 a.m. to 3 p.m.) without sunscreen and with maximum skin exposure; you should do this at least a couple times per week. However, this is not always effective, and there are risks associated with both inadequate and excessive sun exposure.[73]

Therefore, supplementing is often warranted and should be prescribed accordingly to reverse or avoid deficiency. The current RDA for vitamin D for adults is 600 IU per day, although some evidence suggests higher intake may be warranted in certain instances, including deficiency recovery.[74] Since vitamin D is a fat-soluble vitamin (unlike B12), there is a risk of toxicity with larger doses, so we recommend not supplementing blindly. Dosing may also be tricky based on the individual and which form is utilized. Of note, D3 (cholecalciferol) is the natural form and what is formed by the body in response to the sun. D3 is absorbed more effectively than D2 (ergocalciferol). In a 2014 systematic review of vitamin D on mortality, D3 was associated with a decrease in elderly mortality, whereas D2 had no significant beneficial effects.[75] Serum levels fluctuate seasonally with sun availability, so regular monitoring is highly recommended to accurately adjust supplementation needs.

Vitamin K2

Vitamin K, an essential fat-soluble vitamin, is the general classification for several compounds with similar structures, two of which are particularly noteworthy when it comes to diet: phylloquinone (vitamin K1) and menaquinone (vitamin K2). We need these nutrients for blood coagulation, cardiovascular health, and bone metabolism. Phylloquinone is easy to include in one's diet, and abundant in leafy green vegetables, especially collards, spinach, kale, and broccoli. Menaquinone is usually derived from microbial sources and found in fermented foods such as cheese, sauerkraut, and natto (a traditional Japanese food made from soybeans), as well as synthesized via the gut microbiota.[76][77]

According to the Institute of Medicine, adequate adult intake for vitamin K is 120 micrograms for men and 90 micrograms for women.[78] Interestingly, however, most dietary recommendations and food composition tables do not specify which form of K are taken into consideration, and there are no reference daily intakes specifically for K2 yet, so there is a great need for further study and analysis.[79]

Unlike phylloquinone, the intake of menaquinone has been found to profoundly protect the vascular system and, therefore, reduce the risk of cardiovascular disease.[80][81] Menaquinone has also been associated with improved bone health, reduced risk of diabetes, and potentially important roles in immunity, neurological function, multiple cancers, chronic kidney disease, liver disease, and obesity.[82]

Even if you are regularly consuming natto (not all of us love or even have access to it), supplementing with vitamin K2 may be advantageous or even advisable. No adverse effects of vitamin K toxicity are noted for healthy individuals, so it is safe to supplement.[83] However, there is one exception for people who are taking coumarin-based anticoagulant medications (such as warfarin). These drugs require balancing the intake of vitamin K-rich dietary sources and medication dose. These modifications can easily be made with your physician to enable consumption of this important class of nutrients.

Iodine

Iodine is a trace mineral that is necessary for thyroid hormones, metabolism, and neurological development. Sources of iodine vary geographically based on soil conditions and are found primarily in coastal areas. Foods that may contain iodine include sea vegetables and animals that consume concentrated sources of iodine (e.g., fish or animal products secondary to their feed), but the quantities of iodine vary dramatically.[84][85]

While the adult RDA is 150 micrograms per day, iodine deficiency is one of the biggest public health issues globally, impacting approximately one in three people and considered the number one cause of preventable brain damage. It is closely related to goiters, neurocognitive impairment, and cretinism.[86][87] Efforts to address iodine deficiency led to salt iodization programs beginning in the

1920s, which have supplied approximately 70 percent of households throughout much of the world with iodized salt.[88]

Interestingly, many people are not consuming iodized salt because they either avoid salt or opt instead for the ever-expanding assortment of fancy gourmet salt options now available. Since there are limitations on reliable sources of iodine, it is worth considering supplementing to ensure adequate intake.

Zinc

Zinc is an essential trace mineral required for immune function, wound healing, neurological function, and growth. Plant sources include nuts, seeds, legumes (including soyfoods), and whole grains (especially oats). However, the bioavailability of zinc from these foods may be inhibited due to the presence of phytic acid, or phytates, making it less well absorbed than when consumed via animal sources.[89] People on plant-based diets tend to have lower intakes and serum levels of zinc,[90] so implementing strategies such as including foods fortified with zinc or low-dose zinc supplementation can help avoid deficiency. Preparation techniques that reduce the binding of zinc by phytates, such as soaking, sprouting, and leavening (as in bread), can enhance zinc absorption.[91]

Omega-3 Fatty Acids

Omega-3 fat (n-3) is an interesting and complex nutritional issue for plant-based eaters, as well as for anyone who does not consume fish on a regular basis. Although saturated and monounsaturated fats are most commonly discussed, there are only two types of fat that are *essential* in the diet, meaning the body cannot synthesize them endogenously. These polyunsaturated fats include alpha-linolenic acid (ALA), an omega-3 fat, and linoleic acid (LA), an omega-6 fat. Both of these classes of compounds act as precursors to longer-chain polyunsaturated fats, and they serve multiple and opposing functions in the body, including managing inflammation, immunity, hormone production, blood clotting, neurotransmission, and other crucial functions.[92]

ALA is the parent omega-3 compound that our bodies (and the bodies of fish and other animals) can convert into the long-chain eicosapentaenoic acid (EPA) and then further elongate that into docosahexaenoic acid (DHA). We need all these forms for different functions in the body. People on a plant-based diet, or those who do not consume fish for any reason, tend to have lower serum levels of EPA and DHA because no direct source is being consumed.[93] ALA is found in flaxseeds, hempseeds, chia seeds, walnuts, soyfoods, and leafy green vegetables. Whole-plant sources of LA include sesame seeds, tahini, sunflower seeds, pumpkin seeds, corn, wheat germ, and soybeans. But these omega-6 fatty acids are also found ubiquitously in the food supply, mostly as vegetable, seed, and nut oils, which are prevalent in many processed foods that are also low in omega-3 fats.

Because of this, most diets tend to be overly high in omega-6 fats.

A balancing act of these two categories of essential fats becomes paramount, as they have opposing effects and impacts on health. A modern Western diet provides an omega-6:omega-3 ratio of approximately 8:1 to 25:1, while the recommended ratio is closer to 4:1. High intake of omega-6 is associated with a significant reduction in tissue concentrations of EPA and DHA, as it can interfere with the conversion of ALA into EPA and DHA. To avoid the negative health risks associated with an imbalance of omega-6 to omega-3, an emphasis on incorporating more omega-3–rich foods into the diet is key, as is minimizing the intake of processed foods and plant oils and margarines.[94] [95] [96]

In addition, it may be beneficial to include a microalgae-based supplement that includes 200 to 300 milligrams of EPA and DHA.[96] Myriad options are currently available in the marketplace, and they are easy to find. Opting for plant-based versions also helps avoid the associated risks of aggregating heavy metals (such as mercury, lead, and cadmium), industrial pollutants (including DDT, PCBs, and dioxin), and microplastics found in fish and fish oil.[97] [98] [99]

Supplements

That sums up the notable nutrients of right-side triangle eating. As you can see, with just a few considerations, it's quite simple to achieve optimal nutrition with plants. Ultimately, we suggest taking a low-dose multivitamin containing the nutrients discussed previously as well as a microalgae-based formula containing both EPA and DHA. The goal of including these in your regimen is not to replace a healthy diet, as multivitamins will not improve your health nor prevent or treat chronic diseases. Instead, supplements are tools that may help decrease the probability of nutrient inadequacy while minimizing the potential risk of excess.

DAILY AND SEASONAL CHRONOBIOLOGY

Our biology is tied to the day, but is it also driven by the seasons? If you have a backyard or visit a park, do you see anything living that doesn't respond to the seasons? Plants, insects, birds, and squirrels all seem to respond to the seasons without watches, calendars, or computers. These seasonal changes originate with light, temperature, and food. We introduced the concept of *metabolic winter* in Chapter 2 to describe a cool, dark, still, and scarce environment. We hypothesized that these inputs likely trigger our biology in much the same way as they govern the biology in the backyard. On the other hand, *metabolic summer* is dominated by a warm, bright, active, and abundant environment.

Using these two placeholder concepts of metabolic winter and summer, we can reflect on a question: how has modernity impacted these important biological cues? Has it had negative impacts on health? For much of the last century, we've lived

> **" ... eating once or twice a day is biologically normal but perhaps socially extreme. Eating six times a day is biologically extreme and socially normal. "**

in year-round comfortable temperatures with plenty to eat and light on demand. We spend very little time gathering and hunting or seeking shelter. We can find mates with our phones, and it seems robotic companionship is right around the corner. Many of our relationships are with people we've never seen in person. And yet, our brains are still wired much like our ancestors'. If the seven million years of human evolution was represented as a mile, the changes of the last century represent only 0.9 inches. It seems light, temperature, and food still matter.

Meal Frequency

All social interaction revolves around food. We plan our days around standard times for food breaks. We spend nearly the entire day, from wake to sleep, in the fed, or postprandial, state. We eat, the food is digested and absorbed, and the blood's nutrient concentration is increased and returned to normal. This happens at every meal, regardless of size, and as long as the spacing between meals is long enough, blood concentrations return to their normal levels. This is a form of *homeostasis*. In this case, there is a balance between the fed and fasted states that drives much of the metabolic

housecleaning we've described previously. This is why your doctor requests no meals after a certain time the night before surgery; they want to see a true snapshot of your blood panels without a meal interfering. These cycles likely occurred daily in our evolutionary scarce past.

Our ancestors probably didn't have access to enough food to remain in the chronically fed state. Keep in mind that every time we decide to eat, whether it's a Thanksgiving feast or a snack at the coffee pot at the office, this multi-hour process ramps up and down. A host of digestive enzymes (proteins) are synthesized as we described previously, unpacking and packing up genes. The muscles in the stomach and intestinal tract are activated, and there are shifts in blood flow. Digestion is an energy intensive process, and your metabolism ramps up, too. It's not the metabolic boost that fights fat, but rather the metabolic surge that's necessary to handle the digestive action and, importantly, dispose of calories that *can't be stored*. Now think about what happens if one decides to have another snack two hours after having a meal. The blood concentrations from the first meal haven't recovered, and now they are surging up again. And these cycles aren't happening in a vacuum; the timing is important in our overall biological clock.

For most of us, the result is that we remain in the fed state all day long, and if there's a last-minute snack an hour or so before bed, the fed state goes well into your night and sleep process. This is a time when the body temperature actually needs to drop. One of the lesser known roles of melatonin is that it initiates the loss of heat through our extremities so the core and brain temperature can drop, which aids falling asleep.[100] [101] [102] [103] [104] [105] It's one of the reasons hospitals are kept cool for patient rest, as blankets are easily added when necessary. Too much blanketing, especially combined with late-night meals, can both drive up our internal furnaces and trap heat, ultimately disrupting our sleep cycles. When we hear people suggest that they "gain weight when eating late at night," one explanation is eating late is likely less critical than the fact that they spend almost no time in the fasted state.

If we eat just one or two meals a day—a question that Hippocrates pondered 2,400 years ago—and the postprandial state lasts 4 hours for each meal, we stay fed for 4 to 8 hours and conversely fast for the balance of 16 to 20 hours. This is likely a normal human state, but with "intermittent fasting" being among the big fads now, it's as if something special was accomplished. The truth is, eating once or twice a day is biologically normal but perhaps socially extreme. Eating six times a day is biologically extreme and socially normal. In physiological experiments Ray has done for healthspan research and future journal articles, he's spent up to 24 days in medically-supervised, water-only fasts. That may sound like a lot until one recognizes the longest medically supervised water fast was 382 days.[106] Eating once or twice a day isn't some sort

of energy sacrifice, nor should it be any more difficult to do than having a glass of wine on the weekends and not requiring a glass every day. If your energy levels rise and fall that much with a meal, remember, that is habit, not hunger. People feel an abundance of energy weeks into an extended, medically-supervised water fast and don't feel lethargy, headaches, a lack of focus, or irritability. You may, in fact, have habituated to those all-day long frequent meals, and kicking the habit make take a little effort at first.

Our summary on meal frequency is to first avoid using the term "fasting" for anything less than 24 to 36 hours without food or when liquid calories (e.g., juice) is available, as it exaggerates the perceived deprivation. Instead, focus on when you are eating and make those meals—like the ones you'll find in this book—count. If you feel like you're eating for energy or focus, that's more related to missing the habitual cup of coffee than it is a true representation of an energy or nutrient deficit. The most important point here is to avoid eating too late at night due to its circadian impact on sleep and to consider having your first meal (i.e., *break fast*), later in the day and not as soon as you wake. Eating less frequently, particularly keeping right on the Food Triangle, will likely change the size of your meals necessary to stay properly nourished.

The Eyes in Our Eyes

We may have learned in school that rods and cones line the retina in the backs of our eyes. The rods are responsible for low light level vision, while the cones discriminate color in higher light levels. These photoreceptor cells transmit information to the brain through the optic nerve and construct an image of the world.[107] On the way into the brain, the optic nerves also transmit light information to the two small lobes, suprachiasmatic nucleus (SCN), on either side of the almond-sized hypothalamus. If there is a centralized ground zero for homeostasis, the hypothalamus plays a vital role, linking the nervous system with the endocrine system. It produces hormones that signal inhibition or production of other hormones throughout the body. The hypothalamus plays a pivotal role in regulating appetite, thirst, heart rate, blood pressure, electrolyte and fluid balance, digestive tract secretions in the stomach and intestinal tract, sleep, and many other hormonal functions. Together with the pituitary, a pea-sized gland at the base of the brain, and the thyroid, a butterfly-shaped gland in the neck, they form the hypothalamus-pituitary-thyroid axis, or HPT-axis, which constitutes a major feedback for metabolic control as part of the neuroendocrine system.

Consider the rise of depression, fatigue, sleep disorders, or metabolic dysfunction in the last century. How many people do you know, for example, who have a thyroid issue or a sleep disorder? Now, stop to consider our metabolic environment—temperature, light, activity, and food availability—all of these provide input signals and place pressure on the HPT-axis. It is a physiological system that adapted over millions of years to help us survive seasonal adversity. Is it possible that the warm, bright, active, and abundant state of our ubiquitous metabolic summer has created a cascading series of events that, over the decades, may manifest as various forms of metabolic-centric chronic diseases? What we suggested in with our "metabolic winter" hypothesis is that these interdependent systems overlap the cellular biology that also governs longevity.

With this visceral image of the SCN situated atop the hypothalamus, which is in turn communicating with the pituitary and thyroid glands, all within inches of one another, let's return back to the eyes and the impact of daylight and night cycles of the circadian day. In the early 1990s, researchers discovered something amazing while observing mice lacking rods and cones due to a genetic defect: their circadian clocks still responded to light and dark. Despite a century of examining eyes, scientists overlooked a third light-sensitive cell type known as intrinsically photosensitive retinal ganglion cells (ipRGCs).[108] These photoreceptors respond primarily to blue light, and humans who carry a rod and cone genetic defect similar to the mice confirm their existence in us. The ipRGCs dump information about ambient light directly to the SCN, and, as such, are a third eye that has a primary function of syncing our external and internal biological clocks. There are many other hypothesized impacts of these ipRGCs, including links to seasonal affective disorder, migraines, and even improved learning and memory.[109] [110] [111] With the modern-day excessive exposure to light, it may be the brighter blue, especially in the evenings, that is having the most impact on health.[112] Many people now wear blue-blocking sunglasses at night and use special screen colors for laptops, phones, and tablets to cut down the blue frequency.

HEALTH AND OUR BIOLOGICAL CLOCK

We are tied to day and night cycles. In fact, most living organisms—animals, plants, and microbes—have circadian rhythms. Fat accumulation, insulin secretion, insulin sensitivity, immune function, blood pressure, vascular tissue, and food absorption and other intestinal functions are affected by the timing of our circadian clocks.[113] We are affected down to the cellular level, and most of us don't even pay attention to this important biological function.

Pea-Brained Sleep

The pineal gland, a pea-sized gland that sits just behind the hypothalamus, exerts a huge effect on our circadian lives. It's responsible for synthesizing melatonin in direct response to day and night. Melatonin levels begin to rise after sundown (around 8 p.m.) and peak around 3 to 4 a.m. They decline rapidly as we wake and are back to their lowest levels by mid-morning (8–10 a.m.). This pattern is dependent on how our biological time matches up with local time. A teenager (or entrepreneur) staying up late staring into a bright screen can easily shift their biological clock by hours. This results in the alarm clock wake up being much too early in the morning. Independent of when we go to bed, for most, morning begins on schedule, and that's one reason many of us walk around in a constant state of sleep deficit. Poor sleep often arises from a variable bedtime paired with a somewhat inflexible requirement to wake for work or school.

As we age, melatonin synthesis gradually begins to decline (after 40), and sleep patterns become increasingly erratic. Over the last few years, we've worked to increase our sleep, having been early risers all our lives, and now we can routinely sleep for 8 or more hours. Sleep is generally modeled by two processes, the circadian process (process C) and the sleep process (process S). Process C is the general SCN-driven sleep-wake cycle that's related to the biological clocks as we have discussed. Process S is driven by the propensity to fall asleep. It can be generally said that the circadian process (process C) plays an important role in sleep *quantity*, whereas sleep pressure resulting from total time awake (process S) is important for sleep *quality* related to deeper sleep from accumulated sleep debt. We need to stay awake long enough to get high-quality sleep, but our sleep needs to be timed with our circadian clocks to get the maximum quantity of sleep. Both quantity and quality of sleep are important for optimal health.

" Poor sleep often arises from a variable bedtime paired with a somewhat inflexible requirement to wake for work or school. **"**

There are many physiological changes that occur with process C, such as rise and fall in temperature, cortisol (stress hormone) level, and blood pressure. Of course, all of these cycles also have external forces (e.g., light, temperature, and food) that may counter what our bodies are naturally trying to do. For example, body temperature peaks at 5 to 6 p.m. and is the lowest at 5 to 6 a.m. A drop in body temperature is required to fall asleep, and yet so many of us bundle and layer in too many covers causing overheating. This mismatch opposes our circadian hormonal drives. Cooler temperatures in the bedroom and learning to sleep with fewer blankets can be beneficial for people who have difficulty falling asleep or even secondary insomnia (i.e., awakening too early without being able to return to sleep). A cool, dark room is always better, but many have habituated themselves to bright evening TVs, phones, or reading devices and pillow-top, overly warm beds. These can obviously cause issues with SCN and circadian timing release of melatonin and impede the necessary drop in body temperature.

Even if these timings are off a little, the process S sleep drive is based on how long one has been awake and may be enough to doze off. Despite falling asleep easily due to sleep pressure, one may still not get quality sleep (duration and depth), because of these circadian discrepancies. Good sleep hygiene, like diet and activity, requires planning and consistency. Process S is somewhat like a countdown timer that's being continuously restarted. The sleep pressure builds for each hour awake, and like financial debt, it needs to be repaid. It takes time to build up sleep pressure, and it is possible to push through for a while; however, this eventually becomes an issue, and the sleep debt must be eliminated. Given a normal circadian day, we are least alert from 4 to 6 a.m. If you require an alarm clock to wake or tend to sleep later on weekends, then chances are you have some amount of sleep debt. Teenagers not only need a little extra sleep time, but they also tend to be shifted later by a couple of hours as their melatonin rise is typically delayed relative to adults. According to several studies, teenagers aren't fully alert until approximately 10 a.m., which appears to be a result of both a desire to go to bed later combined with a biological need to sleep longer during adolescence.[114] [115] [116] [117] [118]

In general, we are at peak alertness between 6 and 8 p.m. and least alert from 4 to 6 a.m. Daniel P. Cardinali, in *The Educated Brain: Essays in Neuroeducation*, sums up sleep for us,

> Two main, though not mutually exclusive, hypotheses have been predominant in interpreting sleep: (i) sleep is restorative for brain metabolism; (ii) sleep serves memory consolidation and the learning process.

Not only does sleep provide important restorative action for brain metabolism, but it likely assists in a restorative process for overall metabolic health. One can conceptually think of sleep as the mental equivalent of fasting and vice versa. For both sleeping and the fasted state, it's probably not accurate to view these as physiologically dormant states. It's better to think of these as brain and body metabolic revitalization processes. Too little sleep or too much eating could be different sides of the same health coin.

What Time Is It?

How often do you wake up without an alarm clock? Do you sleep longer on the weekend versus a work weekday? These are important first clues to how closely your inner clock is matched to the external world. Let's look at how some of our body functions are governed by the circadian clock. Starting at the left at 6 a.m., we begin a 24-hour biological cycle. One way to determine how your external and internal clocks match is to assess what time you wake up naturally without an alarm clock. About two hours before that time is one way researchers assess the beginning of your biological day. This time is when your body reaches its lowest core temperature in the day.

Many physiological processes, such as core body temperature, bowel movements, blood pressure, alertness, and cardiovascular efficiency, follow a repeatable circadian rhythm. It's hard to believe all of this is controlled by these circadian clocks, and that your

environment is key to driving these changes at the appropriate time. Not only this, but there is a strong link between the sirtuins and the circadian clock as well. [119] [120] [121]

WIGGLING AND SHIVERING FOR HEALTH

There is little doubt that exercise offers advantages across the lifespan and throughout the systems of the body, including cardiometabolic, neuromuscular, cellular, musculoskeletal, psychological, and more. While it is not completely understood how exercise impacts longevity, it appears to be related to similar protective hormesis, as seen with dietary restriction.

One puzzling reaction to increased activity is the production of a hormone, irisin, which paradoxically increases a special kind of fat tissue, brown adipose tissue (BAT).[122] This brown adipose tissue is interesting in that it's loaded with those mitochondrial power plants, giving it the reddish-brown color, and its purpose is to generate waste heat from fat. Irisin is a protein named after Iris, the Greek goddess and messenger to the Olympian gods. Irisin is believed to signal another protein, peroxisome proliferator-activated receptor gamma coactivator 1-alpha (PGC-1α), which is the master regulator of mitochondrial (the cellular power plant) biogenesis (creation of energy). PGC-1α boosts the DNA production of two important cellular functions: producing new mitochondria (mitochondrial biogenesis) and cellular remodeling (e.g.,

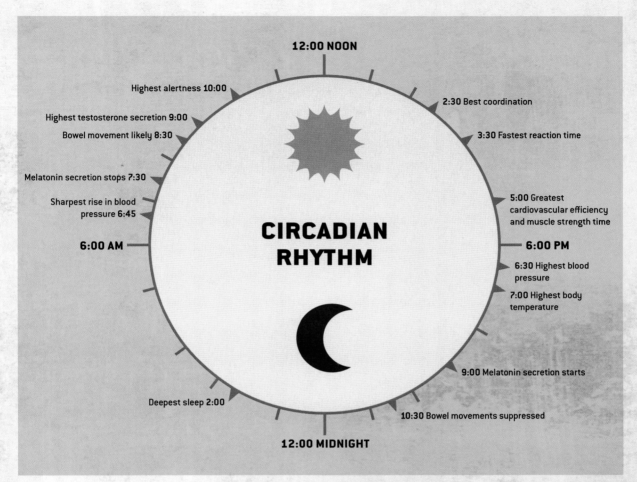

Circadian clocks govern many processes in the body and may significantly contribute to the accumulation of age-related chronic disease.

transforming white adipose tissue to the thermally active, energy-hungry brown adipose tissue).[123] [124] [125]

Our "metabolic winter" hypothesis was centered on the idea that cold, exercise, fasting, and oxidative stress all trigger PGC-1α and are major signaling pathways studied in longevity. What's puzzling is that exercise, the expenditure of energy presumably to meet some evolutionary need to find food, fight, or flee, would signal irisin, a protein that modifies energy storage fat cells to become waste-heat generating tissue (BAT). Fasting or a fasting-mimicking diet can also trigger the same wasteful heat-generating tissue. Why would starving and wiggling produce a tissue designed to waste energy stores to produce heat? What cellular advantage might be conferred by this combination of signaling by exercise, cold, and fasting?

One explanation is that some of the benefits from exercise originate through exercise-mimicking shivering, the first biological step in combating mild cold stress. Dietary restriction without malnutrition seems to provide some of the benefits of fasting without actually fasting. Likewise, exercise may trigger some of the evolutionary benefits of mild cold stress adaptive mechanisms without actually shivering.[126] [127] Could one health benefit of exercise be that it serves to mimic shivering? When we are exposed to mild cold stress, the initial response is to shiver. During shivering, the waste heat generated through involuntary activation of rapid muscular contraction helps to warm the body. Does exercise mimic this primitive survival response? It's interesting that shivering resulting from mild cold exposure is often replaced by a non-shivering generation of heat via BAT. When we measure this shiver/non-shiver transition in the lab, we see a shift from glucose, the fuel of explosive moves and most exercise, to fat.

Keep in mind that lifting weights, biking, or running increases strength or performance through the breakdown of tissue during the activity. That stress, in turn, acts through hormesis to signal the rebuilding of the tissue with increased performance (hypertrophy). If one is in metabolic winter—cool, dark, still, and scarce (food)—breaking down tissue during a nutritional deficit might negatively impact the repair process,

whereas generating the heat directly through activating BAT might avoid shivering and tissue breakdown altogether. While it's common to believe that exercise preserves tissue during dieting, the differences are very minor.[128]

On the other hand, it makes much more evolutionary sense that the body prioritizes fat over brain, organ, or muscle tissue in times of no food. In this winter survival mode, perhaps these direct cellular, heat-generating adaptations are merely a way to preserve us in a time of scarcity. BAT can generate heat more efficiently than shivering by cellular level changes that don't require the middle movement step. Together, fasting, cold stress, and exercise may act synergistically to generate heat by inducing a cellular-level mechanism that creates heat without the potential damage of the prolonged muscular contraction. This maximizes heat production, sources the fuel from fat stores, and minimizes the possibility for tissue breakdown.

STAY ACTIVE, LIVE LONG

With respect to general well-being over the long run, movement helps to protect bone density and cardiovascular endurance, minimize muscle loss, and maintain flexibility and balance. Those in the longest-lived populations were active, but were not running extreme races or spending hours in a gym. They moved, lifted, pushed, pulled, and engaged in activities of daily living. However, one does not need to scale mountains or flip cars to achieve these benefits. In fact, tapering movement into a more casual, less intensive intention might be optimal over the long run. Avoiding injury is also crucial for sustainability and long-term health, so a lighter fitness regimen is likely just right for the general population.

Some examples of how to apply movement include:

- Using an activity or step counter to aim for 10,000 or more steps per day.
- Engaging in active social meetings (hiking or walking instead of meeting at a restaurant).
- Stretching a bit in a yoga class or simply at home.
- Light strength training with weights or your own body weight.
- Playing a game of tennis or golf with a friend, taking a dance class, or swimming.
- Parking farther from the office or store and taking the stairs.

In closing, there is no doubt that we are inextricably linked to the day-night cycle, and a mismatch could very well contribute to out-of-control eating binges. Diet and activity level that mimics those times of metabolic winter, perhaps the peaceful calm before the storm, are quickly overcome by the excesses of metabolic spring, summer, and fall. It's likely in some evolutionary past that the abundance of metabolic summer provided for excessive amino acids that led to increased fecundity (reproductive rates), but today we live in a world of metabolic summer abundance year-round. Also, one can imagine that the seasonal photo period has been destroyed with the ability to pollute our circadian clocks using late night lights and screens.

Are we surprised that the rise of chronic disease could potentially be partly fueled by living for decades in the year-round excesses of metabolic summer's warm, bright, active, and abundant? We think it is fascinating just how much our health and the health of others has been improved by periods of a few months of increased cool (not cold) temperatures, sleep, and dietary restriction. We may need to take a little break from the never-ending physiological demands of hyperactivity dressed up as athletic competition. Likewise, we probably need a time of reduced food intake without malnourishment both to deplete our stores a little, and, more importantly, to activate those evolutionary survival genes that seem to convey longevity and healthspan in many biological species. Winter never comes, and perhaps your health depends on taking a few months to repair, rejuvenate, and refresh with a little less food, warmth, and activity. Less is more in healthspan.

"… perhaps your health depends on taking a few months to repair, rejuvenate, and refresh with a little less food, warmth, and activity."

HEALTHSPAN HABITS

With much of the *why* out of the way, the question now becomes *how*. How do we implement all of the history and science lessons we've covered into our daily lives and give it our best go? This is a question scientists, researchers, and healthcare professionals have been attempting to answer since the beginning of recorded history. It is represented by the tale of the fountain of youth, the hope-filled search for some mythical source that could halt our mortality so that we could appreciate our health and vitality with our accumulated wisdom.

Beyond the rapid potential successes being attempted in the lab with pharmaceuticals, what can we each do, on an individual level, considering the information and tools we have at our fingertips right now?

This list of **10 Healthspan Habits** is a summary of our conclusions on how to translate the science into action.

1. **DON'T BE DRIVEN BY DIET DOGMA.** Avoid the woes and downward spirals of macroconfusion by recognizing it in the trends and maintaining your focus on foods. If you stumble upon an article or a news report about "a new diet" or "a superfood" or "toxic ingredients," stop and dig deeper before making any decisions. If it sounds too good (or bad) to be true, it probably is. Remember that the preponderance of evidence on nutrition over time has not changed by much. Herein lies the problem, and it becomes a mix of the telephone game and unearned expertise. Keep your language centered on whole foods— "eat carrots" versus "eat low-glycemic, complex carbohydrates."

2. **KEEP EATING RIGHT.** Use the Food Triangle as a model to visualize and remember how different diets work. An emphasis on the right side of the triangle, particularly the foods at the top, enables the consumption of the most health-promoting nutrients (e.g., dietary fiber and phytonutrients) while avoiding excessive amounts of chronic disease-promoting compounds (e.g., excessive essential amino acids, heme iron, saturated fat, etc.) and the chronic overnutrition brought about by bottom feeding.

3. **EAT LESS.** Nutrition is not an emergency and your metabolism won't break with time off from swallowing. The only way we have ever extended healthspan and lifespan with diet in nearly every organism tested thus far—in the lab as well as in the few populations that have demonstrated success when analyzed—is with dietary restriction without malnutrition. To achieve this goal:

   » Eat vegetables, fruits, whole grains, legumes, mushrooms, nuts, seeds, herbs, and spices to gain the most nutritional bang for your caloric buck.

   » Eat less frequently.

   » Eat less volume.

4. **OBSERVE "RARE AND APPROPRIATE."** Be mindful of people and places rather than time between events when it comes to decisions of decadence. What and how you eat *most* of the time matters overall. Rather than building in "cheat days," allow yourself to have an R&A when eating with someone meaningful to you or when visiting a unique place. There aren't any data suggesting diet must be perfect, but even if you try to be perfect, you probably won't be. Our food choices are created through habit, so attempt to stay on plan. It takes time for the new normal to set in place, so strive to reserve those deviations for truly special occasions.

5. **SUPPLEMENT AS NEEDED.** We suggest a low-dose multivitamin containing vitamins B12, D, and K2 and the minerals iodine and zinc. We also suggest a microalgae-based, long-chain omega-3 fatty acid supplement that includes both EPA and DHA.

6. **BE ACTIVE.** The opposite of sedentary is active, not exercise. Focus on movement and activity, not only intensive exercise. Stand while speaking on the phone, park a little farther away from the store, take the stairs, and increase leisure activities with friends and family. There is benefit to the stress from intensive activity, but all too often, this may be mitigated by overnutrition, whether the excessive intake need is perceived or real, which likely mitigates the activity with negative impacts in excessive diets. Remember, organisms subjected to dietary restriction without malnutrition perform better on physical tasks, but excessive activity doesn't compensate for a bad diet.

7. **OPTIMIZE CHRONOBIOLOGY.** Optimize your circadian clock with proper sleep hygiene. Thirty minutes of bright light in the morning will help anchor your circadian clock. In the evening, pay more attention to the sun variations in the light outside. Turn off screens at least an hour before bed. Go to sleep in a dark, cool room and don't use excessive blankets. Melatonin supplementation may be helpful for you, particularly if you're over 40, and it also seems to be a strong sirtuin activator.

8. **INCORPORATE MILD COLD STRESS.** "Gloves before sweaters will make you look better." Practice layering for skiing in reverse. Take your layers *with* you, not *on* you. Cover your cold symptoms (hands, ears, face, and feet) and leave your torso exposed. Lower the thermostat a little. Mild cold stress doesn't require ice baths: think *cool* not cold. Perform a contrast shower—cycling 10 seconds of warm water followed by 20 seconds of cold water, and repeat that cycle 10 times, ending on cold. You'll feel refreshed and awake in the morning, and it will make falling asleep far easier at night.

9. **EXPLORE OCCASIONAL FASTING.** Our brains don't shut down when we sleep, and it seems well accepted that critical housekeeping activities occur during this altered state. Our metabolism also doesn't shut down during extended times refraining from swallowing. Your metabolic DVR may be full. Take some time to binge-watch those meals you already ate to make some room for next season's excitement. Spending a weekend by swallowing only water allows for cellular and metabolic house cleaning to occur. It's foolish to believe we are managing our physiology through purposeful swallowing. We mostly do it for entertainment, and the results are self-evident if you'll take the time to look around. There are myriad advantages of fasting that are worth exploring further. Of course, make sure you discuss this with your healthcare provider first.

10. **CREATE MINDFUL MOMENTS.** Make arrangements every day for unstructured time. Some meditate, while others might just vegetate. No matter your method, counting every minute is a great way to squander laughter, joy, smiles, love, wonder, amazement, and meaning on accounting. You're never going to be done. For some, this will mean waking up a little earlier without jumping on social media and email, and for others, it will mean taking some time in the day to unplug. Don't let others dominate your priority list because health will almost surely be the first item to fall off completely. There's always an excuse to eat off plan, but keep in mind it's not mandatory to share a swallow to have deep and meaningful connections with those around you.

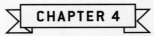

FLAVORS, FALLACIES, AND FOOD FANTASIES

CONVENIENT, FAMILIAR, AND ENJOYABLE

Did you buy this book to make a change? Perhaps it was a gift. Perhaps you're already dealing with some sort of health crisis or trying to avoid one. Food is highly social, and therein lies the challenge. Making a change requires time and tenacity. Maybe you're already exclusively eating plants and you need to cut down on the plant-sourced junk food. Maybe you eat too much salt or can't turn on the stove without a bottle of olive oil in your hand. Perhaps you haven't cooked before. Some might panic at the question, "wait, you don't eat cheese?"

Everyone starts somewhere, and changing habits requires time—*uninterrupted time*—to find that "new normal" we discussed in Chapter 1. Remember, until your new diet is equally convenient, familiar, and enjoyable to your old one, you don't have a choice; one or more of these will likely dominate your plate. We want to make that as easy as possible. Food and cooking can be so pretentious. They can be divisive, too, if you stray too far from the norm. Unless you always eat alone, you're likely to interact with another person, and their own favorite foods and habits often get piled onto your plate. Some of our recipes are crowd pleasers, independent of your current diet, while some might seem bland if you've recently switched from a hyperpalatable diet with excessive sugar, salt, and oil.

LESSONS FROM THE LUNCH BUNCH

If you're making a decision alone about what to eat for lunch at the office, you are completely flexible in terms of lunch time, cuisine, and cost. When you invite someone to eat with you, the decision about eating becomes a little more complicated. Add the third, fourth, and fifth person, and you'll soon find yourself standing in the hall trying to figure out how to meet everyone's needs. From a distance, the entire discussion seems like a silly first-world problem, despite people having strong opinions about what, where, and when to eat. We tend to overthink these decisions because we live with the modern luxury to do so. If you're trying to make a change, it will be easier on your own. You may need to eat a recipe a few times or revisit one after a few weeks or months of eating this way, as your tastes will change over time. New habits can be formed. You will find your new favorite foods, but it won't likely happen until after the old food has been off the plate for some time. Cheat days are for cheaters, not winners. This is likely why people who make diet changes for ideological reasons are successful, as their belief system helps them push through to new habits and joy.

> " You will find your new favorite foods, but it won't likely happen until after the old food has been off the plate for some time. Cheat days are for cheaters, not winners. "

For evidence of just how crazy our world is, have you ever looked down 75 linear feet of shelf space at the grocery store searching for the perfect pet food *flavor*? Do starving cats and dogs care what flavor they are eating? Pets can also develop finicky habits, and we alone are responsible for those habits. We're also completely responsible for their resulting weight issues and chronic disease. A truly hungry person or pet will eat what's available. Headaches, lethargy, lack of focus, and irritability aren't symptoms of hunger. They are similar to the physiological responses we experience when we suddenly remove habitually ingested things like coffee, alcohol, or tobacco. Most of our clients experience these symptoms in the first weeks of diet change. After a short while, the symptoms fade and they find joy in their new food.

We need to internalize the idea that eating a diet of vegetables, fruits, whole grains, legumes, mushrooms, nuts, seeds, herbs, and spices is a modern-day *luxury* of human agricultural prowess. For millennia, humans ate whatever they could find to survive. While everyone wants to look back for ancestral clues about what was eaten, that information doesn't say much about the kind of diet that will reduce chronic disease after ages 45 to 50, when evolution is mostly done with us. Today, we have an incredible degree of choice, even in the smallest town's market. Most of us squander the choice by meeting our hedonistic palate desires. Everybody will die of something, one might suggest. But how many of those

people will say the same thing and refuse treatment when their chronic disease lottery ticket is drawn early in life? They'll take medicine that makes them nauseous. They'll submit themselves to radiation treatment or surgically remove body parts. After disease hits, they sometimes submit to a temporary near-death hell to stay alive. Even though there's ample research that dietary restriction without malnutrition over a lifetime would likely delay or completely mitigate premature age-related chronic disease, most won't make small changes now to avoid drastic, less effective actions tomorrow. We want you to reconsider this with care.

As we state at the start of this book, we are emphatic in our assertion that eating this healthspan diet will not make you immortal. However, we are confident that eating on the right side of the Food Triangle, with limited food adulterants, will likely increase your healthspan. This will require the acquisition of new palate pleasures and new food habits. We believe there's a starting point in this book for *everyone*. Clearly, some recipes will be superior to others because we all start with different food habits; however, there is a soup, salad, side, and sweet in this book for you.

RECLAIMING YOUR PALATE

It's going to take a while to develop a new palate. Even during the testing of recipes for this book, there were discussions on too little salt or too much of something else. One problem with culinary school is that it teaches everyone to cook like a restaurant chef. For us, the food at restaurants—especially restaurants that exclusively serve plants—is often much too salty, oily, and sweet. We still like it, but we now feel the meal beyond the "I ate too much" sensation. Typically, salt drives excessive thirst later that evening and the next day. We feel puffy and, in one case, after Julieanna was shooting a series in New York City for 10 days, Ray became hypertensive for the first time in his life from daily dining out.

THE FIVE TASTES

We sense flavor with both taste and smell. Remember the grade school image of the tongue with sweet, salt, sour, and bitter in zones on the tip, sides, and back? Well, forget that; it's wrong.[1] We learned in the early 2000s that the tiny, onion-shaped taste buds, even smaller than the bumpy papillae you see on your tongue, are composed of four types of cells; singularly and in combination, they sense the various basic flavors. The good news is that what you learned about the basic four flavors is still correct. Sweet and salty make things delicious, and we seem to develop a flavor affinity for sour and bitter along the way. We also should introduce a fifth taste, *umami,* the savory, rich flavor found in meat, fish, aged cheeses, and mushrooms.

One challenge with describing these five flavors is that they are often conflated with something else. A ripe banana is sweet, but it also tastes like bananas. Capers are salty, but they taste like capers. When considering the five flavors, it might be helpful to identify them in their pure forms. Once you have a firm grasp on these, it becomes much easier to know how to adjust your food.

Considered in their pure forms, we would list the following ingredients:

Sweet - sucrose (table sugar)
Salty - sodium chloride (table salt)
Sour - acetic acid (white vinegar)
Bitter - quinine (used in tonic water)
Umami - monosodium glutamate (MSG)

Scientists hypothesize that each of these flavors served an evolutionary advantage. For example, umami allows detection of amino acids in food; sweet is an indication of glucose energy content; sour may warn of fermented or spoiled food; and bitter is associated with potentially toxic substances. All the science aside, food companies and restaurants know that these flavors drive our appetites and subsequently, sales. It's easy to make food taste amazing if one cranks up the hyperpalatability volume. However, as you might have guessed, that's not the easiest path to increasing healthspan. Those fried, salty, sweet, and savory appetizers aren't called de-appetizers for good reason. Eating more before dinner means eating more at dinner, too. The

"The fundamental urge to excessively swallow decadent food had sound biological reason in a world of scarcity."

FOOD AND FLAVOR

	TASTE	TASTE SUBSTANCE	COMMON FOODS
	Sweet	Sucrose Fructose Glucose	Sugar Honey Candy
	Sour	Acetic acid Citric acid Lactic acid	Vinegar Lemons Limes Yogurt
	Salty	Sodium chloride	Salt
	Bitter	Caffeine Alcohol Momordicin	Coffee Bitter melon Chocolate (90% cacao mass)
	Umami	Glutamate Inosinate Guanylate	Tomatoes Cheese Meat Fish Dried shiitake mushrooms

fundamental urge to excessively swallow decadent food had sound biological reason in a world of scarcity. When we stumbled upon food, it was wise to eat as much as we could. It's those urges to consume massive quantities that we need to tame a bit. We must enter a pact together. With a few small compromises, we'll crank our food up a notch from the bland-and-boring recipes found in many health-focused cookbooks, and you need to tame your tastebuds to the normal levels for nature's appetizing flavors.

It might be obvious from our frugivorous primate first cousins that our quest for sweet is likely driven by fruit and other sweet and starchy foods. It seems sugar is an almost universally vilified food component. We have many copies of the salivary amylase gene, AMY1. It creates the protein enzyme, amylase, that breaks down starches to simple sugar.[2] Is our love for sweet nature or nurture? Our first cues to innate taste drives come from infancy. When neonates are exposed to the five basic flavors, only two come out on top: sweet and umami.[3]

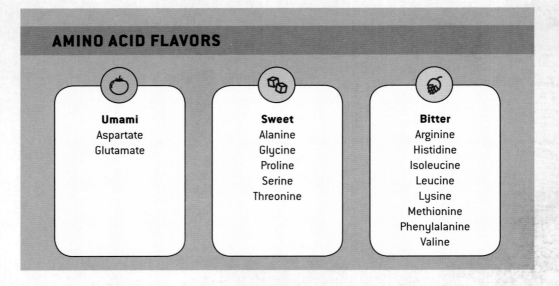

AMINO ACID FLAVORS

Umami
Aspartate
Glutamate

Sweet
Alanine
Glycine
Proline
Serine
Threonine

Bitter
Arginine
Histidine
Isoleucine
Leucine
Lysine
Methionine
Phenylalanine
Valine

Researchers looked at facial expressions, such as nose wrinkling, lip pursing, and gaping in reaction to different flavors and recorded the responses. Sweet causes lip smacking and sucking. And then there was umami. When the babies were given a dilute vegetable broth, the response was similar to the other flavors, but when glutamate was added to the broth, it elicited the same smacking and sucking response as sweet. The explanation for this probably comes from analysis of human breast milk, but we need a quick science sidetrack on glutamate because myths about MSG are pervasive. Oh, I feel the headache.

Umami was discovered and named in 1907 by Japanese scientist Kikunae Ikeda of Tokyo Imperial University (now the University of Tokyo).[4] Professor Ikeda noticed that a taste common in Japanese *dashi*, a seaweed broth, that did not fit into the traditional sweet, salty, sour, and bitter categories. He isolated the main amino acid component in kombu dashi to be glutamate. A year later, in 1908, he patented the separation process, and formed Anjinomoto, which still operates today.[5] [6] Other Japanese scientists later discovered two more umami-containing DNA building block nucleotides, disodium inosinate (IMP) from fish and disodium guanylate (GMP) from mushrooms.[7] We've learned a great deal about umami in the last century. Despite umami's important role in cooking around the world, it is still much less understood in the West from a pure flavor perspective. Umami may be unnecessarily limited or missing in many plant-centric, right-side Food Triangle meals.

Umami: Sensing Amino Acids

Amino acids are the building blocks of thousands of proteins. A subset of these, indispensable or essential amino acids, originates only from diet for humans and other animals. Plants make all 20 amino acids because most plants can't eat. When the total protein content of food is discussed, the specificity of amino acid content is missed, and that drives macroconfusion. Free amino acids exist in every cell and in the vascular system, ready for protein synthesis should cellular DNA and other regulatory mechanisms give the call for more insulin, hemoglobin, amylase, or keratin (all proteins). Cells—plant and animal alike—destroy and synthesize many thousands of different proteins every day; some proteins last only seconds. What if those free amino acids that vary in concentration had a flavor of their own? What if you could sense them? Beyond terrorizing babies with bitter food,

scientists have also tested human response to the 20 amino acids.

As it turns out, they primarily fall into three categories of flavor: bitter, sweet, and umami.[8][9] Most of the dietary essential amino acids are bitter, but at least one is sweet (threonine). The real surprise here is the two responsible for umami. Aspartate and glutamate are both internally synthesized by our bodies, and we don't need to obtain them from diet. Glutamine is one of the most abundant amino acids in nature. It can exist in several forms that are more or less metabolically equivalent, but it's best known in its ionic form, glutamate. How important is it? It's by far the most concentrated free amino acid in human breast milk, and likely why a newborn reacts so positively to it.[10]

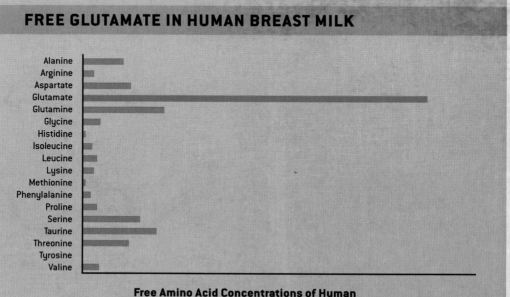

FREE GLUTAMATE IN HUMAN BREAST MILK

Alanine
Arginine
Aspartate
Glutamate
Glutamine
Glycine
Histidine
Isoleucine
Leucine
Lysine
Methionine
Phenylalanine
Proline
Serine
Taurine
Threonine
Tyrosine
Valine

**Free Amino Acid Concentrations of Human
Breast Milk at One-Month Infant Age**

It seems umami plays a powerful role in human flavor. Glutamate can be concentrated in many foods. It's why sun-dried tomatoes and tomato paste add such an amazing flavor to recipes. It's the flavor that emerges as Parmesan cheese ages. This is not a compound similar to MSG—it is absolutely identical. As it turns out, the MSG panic dates back to 1968 and a single 358-word letter to the editor written by Robert Ho Man Kwok, MD, Senior Research Investigator, National Biomedical Research Foundation and published in the *New England Journal of Medicine*.[11] This letter spawned 50 years of debate, research, and worldwide strong opinions, but there wasn't enough evidence then or now to raise such a strong response.[12] There are even studies that suggest benefits to MSG. Comprehensive reviews looking at clinical trials over the last half century suggest concerns about MSG are far more likely to be perceived issues than real ones.[13]

Why does it matter? Should you grab a shaker of MSG? That's not our message. When we examine food and taste across a wide section of cultures, umami seems to be an important element of food and enjoyment. Glutamate is not only found in breast milk, but also in a wide range of vegetables like onions, garlic, soy beans, carrots, celery, corn, green peas, and potatoes. Glutamate dominates umami in certain foods like tomatoes, miso, kimchi, and Parmesan cheese, but there are additional important umami flavor molecules. The nucleotides GMP and IMP have a similar impact on umami perception in food. IMP is found in fish, chicken, pork, beef, and nori (seaweed). GMP is found in shiitake mushrooms (see Magic Mushroom Powder, page 242), dried tomatoes, and nori. GMP and IMP work synergistically in the chicken stock of Chinese cooking, the beef and chicken stock of Western soups, and the dashi (kombu seaweed and bonito) of Japanese soups to enhance flavor. We demonstrate umami in the cooking classes we teach, and everyone is absolutely shocked at how much it impacts flavor. It seems unlikely that something with such a profound effect on flavor would not be evolutionarily important.

There are many ways to get sweet, salty, sour, and bitter into our healthspan diet, but umami stands alone in its unique flavor pocket, and it makes a huge difference in food around the world. MSG has been vilified, but it may still have a role, if for no other reason than for people to understand and perceive umami flavor. As we will see in the next section on food adulterants, it might also be a way for some to ramp up flavor without reaching for the salt shaker.

Food Adulterants:
When, What, Why, and How Much?

When using the Food Triangle, we emphasize *whole* foods, as they provide nutrition and energy. There is an additional category of ingredients that are added to foods for purposes other than nourishment, including to modify texture, flavor, shelf stability, color, thickening, and more. Perhaps the most commonly used ingredients in the kitchen that flirt within the boundaries of this group are sugars, oils, and salt. While each of these can be used for nutriment, they tend to be overused in myriad ways to push food flavor over the top. When used in excess, these can create health issues. Not only is there widespread controversy on the use of these items, but there are also varying examples of their purpose throughout recorded history. In times of economic scarcity, sugars, oils, and salt helped enhance consumption of affordable, available, and low-calorie food to support survival. In modern times of food abundance, these items are used in excess to create hyperpalatable, empty-calorie food, encouraging overconsumption and overnutrition.

So how much is enough? Which ones do we use and why? We agree that our palates become desensitized to these basic flavor sensations with increased use, which may drive us to eat and to desire more. Some paint this situation as a sugar addiction, but there's another way to think about these flavor habits. We are much more adept at detecting change in flavor than we are at detecting the actual level of that flavor. The same is true for temperature when coming inside on a warm or cool day. The house may feel overly hot or cold to you, yet comfortable to those already inside. Likewise, your perception of flavor is dependent on how you eat most days. When we return from travels in Thailand or China, it takes a couple of weeks for our salt detection to become more sensitive because it's hard to escape the cultural significance of salt in those countries.

We recommend whenever possible to use whole-food sources of the basic flavors. For example, we use dates and grapes to create sweetness. White grapes are often relatively neutral in flavor, and when they are at the peak sweetness, they can be frozen in a freezer bag and used to sweeten other foods. (Our Poppy Seed Dressing on page 234 is an example.) Again, there is a limit; sometimes, the grape or date flavor is too strong, and it may be necessary to use another sweetener. In some cases, a teaspoon of sugar won't help the medicine go down, but rather make a healthy, average dish amazing and keep you on plan to avoid the medicine altogether.

In our cooking, we also sweeten with molasses and maple syrup. Because both have a flavor other than sweetness, they naturally limit how much one can use without these additional flavors dominating the dish. Molasses, the byproduct of refined sugar production, also contributes an umami component, as it has a 0.3 to 0.5 percent glutamate concentration. Maple syrup has a more neutral flavor, but it does have distinct characteristics. The same is true with dates, which fall somewhere between these two. When possible, add fresh fruit to the dressing or sauce as a first choice for sweetness.

The Slippery Slope with Oil

As we described in the section on oxidative priority, excess fat in the diet becomes stored, primarily due to overall excessive meal volume and frequency. We are in the "fed" state too often.

Oil is one of the food adulterants that is easy to use in excess, and it provides empty calories that are easy to store. From a culinary sense, beyond a certain point, using oil just adds calories with no palate upside. In our kitchen, we don't cook with oil. More specifically, we don't start every recipe with the addition of lard, bacon grease, coconut oil, or olive oil to the pan or dish. We don't use oil or cooking spray oils to prevent sticking in pans; it's not necessary. We don't fry vegetables submerged in oil, whereby their natural water content is replaced by fat. These cooking techniques had a place when food was economically scarce, but today, they are often carried through in cooking by tradition, not necessity. Instead, we tend to use whole-food sources of fats in sauces and dressings. As we have seen in the case of sweet and salty, there are limits to this approach from a culinary perspective.

In that sense, we use various flavored oils, particularly chili, toasted sesame, and robust olive oils, as adjunct flavors in teaspoon quantities. This approach more closely resembles the use of a robust herb, such as basil or rosemary, than how one might traditionally use oil. The oleogustus ("fatty taste") quality of oil is also related to mouthfeel, and it acts as a carrier for complex flavors so they can be detected. It is amazing how far a teaspoon of oil will go in enhancing flavor without compromising health and, pun intended, not be the slippery slope to television-food-show, home-cooked, junk food recipes. We've taken the time to use the minimum amount, and we do so in a way that will maximize your perception of these for impactful flavor.

The ingredient police are everywhere. You know them, and they take every opportunity to bash this or that ingredient. We want you to be more relaxed about this and know that practicing "rare and appropriate" will go a long way in making your transformation a success. When salt, sugar, oil, or MSG are used to make junk food hyperpalatable, this is unquestionably a bad idea. Using ill-defined labels such as *natural*, *organic*, or *processed* confuses the issue even more. On the other hand, when these food adulterants are used infrequently and *in limited quantities* to make healthy food taste amazing, they can be a powerful tool in the pantry.

USING FLAVOR ENHANCEMENT

Let's address how we might enhance flavor without decreasing the healthspan benefits of eating right on the Food Triangle. Remember, these food adulterants, even the demonized MSG, aren't acutely toxic. Most of the negative association comes from their frequent use to make empty calories hyperpalatable. We want to focus very specifically on four elements of flavor enhancement: sweet, salty, oily (oleogustus), and umami. For the most part, sour (citrus, vinegar, etc.) and bitter aren't the salient ingredients for empty calorie junk food. These components nearly always must be

> **"How much of a substance is in each bite isn't the only thing to consider. How *many* bites is often far more important."**

balanced out with other flavors to reach the tip of gluttonous behavior.

When thinking about flavor enhancement, our first goal should be an attempt to accomplish this with the whole-food ingredients. For example, celery has a salty flavor, but it also has a distinct flavor of celery. Can one increase the salty flavor without overpowering the dish with celery? When one considers our Simple Stock (page 96), we include carrots and celery, as these both add a complex salty flavor. In addition, there is sweetness from the carrots, complex aromatics and sweetness of the onion, umami from the shiitake, and background flavor from the bay leaves. Celery can be used to add salt, to a point, but beyond that, the recipe may require an adjunct salt additive. Next, one might turn to something like tamari, which is a more concentrated additive of salt than celery, but it, too, has other flavors from the fermented soy. It might not be a good choice for every recipe, but it adds an element of umami and salt, while still being easy to measure.

We want you to make sound decisions and enjoy your food because that will lead to consistency and permanent lifestyle transformation. How much of a substance is in each bite isn't the only thing to consider. How *many* bites is often far

more important. The primary problem we face is likely chronic overnutrition. A secondary issue is that food adulterants are used in quantities many times greater than you'll see in this book to make empty calorie foods appear decadent. Even fructose, the often maligned isomer of glucose, sprinkled on a not-quite-ripe peach isn't the same as drinking a 32-ounce soda sweetened with high-fructose corn syrup. And it's not only the high-fructose corn syrup that's at issue; the empty calories are a bigger concern than the scary high-fructose corn syrup name. There isn't a bright line here, but most people readily understand the difference between junk food and whole food, particularly if they don't use the macroconfusion labels of protein, carbohydrate, or fat. We want you to explore using food adulterants in a minimal way to *enhance healthy food* without becoming excessive. If you don't use them and are happy, that's okay, too. If you think food adulterants are excessive in your diet, often the best way to begin is to drop them altogether for some period of adjustment. Then add back with purpose, not excess.

Oil

We aren't going to address weight loss or weight gain, and we assume you're not grabbing the bottle of olive oil while turning on the stovetop. We've tried to be clear that we use oils in a culinary sense like one would use rosemary or basil. Even within the plant-based community, there are battles taking place between the fat-avoiders, oil-includers, and moderation-seekers. People argue *passionately* for one side or another. Our advice is to avoid cooking with oil. Use it for the culinary flavor or texture instead of as a primary caloric ingredient. In general, one should limit added oil to about 1 teaspoon per serving, and it should have a purpose. You'll see a few recipes in this book with chili oil, olive oil, and toasted sesame oil. In most recipes that call for olive oil, it can easily be skipped.

Here's a trick to use oil in a way to get the most out of the least—use it *after* you cook. Steam or cook your vegetables or food with water to maximize the water content, and add oil at the very end. Since oil and water are immiscible, the oil won't soak into the vegetables and it will be the first thing to hit your tongue. If you've ever wondered why steamed vegetables at Chinese restaurants taste so amazing, it's because they are often quickly blanched in oil before they're steamed. This leaves a very light coating on the surface, but doesn't drive the oil into the vegetable like frying. An even better approach when using a culinary oil that will impart both a mouthfeel and a flavor is to add it at the end of cooking. This will ensure the minimum quantity is used for the maximum flavor benefit. Additionally, when sautéing garlic, consider doing it toward the end of cooking using a teaspoon of oil in the center of the wok or pan. The garlic flavor will be concentrated and carried onto the surface of the food with the very thin film of oil (see Spicy Sesame Asparagus Aubergine, page 205).

Salt

Perceived salt flavor is highly variable, and it's possible to habituate to high and low amounts. The American Heart Association suggests a daily intake target of 1,500 milligrams of sodium and not to exceed 2,300 milligrams. To put that in perspective, one teaspoon of salt contains 2,325 milligrams of sodium—and that's before we put it on anything. Keep in mind that many items, particularly vegetable broth and canned foods, may contain significant added sodium. It's in sauces and condiments as well. Even when trying to limit sodium, it's very easy for it to become excessive. We've discussed the use of salty condiments such as tamari or soy sauce, but no matter the source, when added right before serving, it creates the most salty flavor impact.

Consider that the two slices of bread to make a sandwich contain more sodium than a single serving of potato chips. It doesn't seem possible, but here's why: the bread has the salt baked into it, whereas the potato chips are fried and therefore saturated with oil. Salt doesn't dissolve in the oil and sits on the surface to hit your tongue as the chip touches. We can use this to our advantage—if one is adding a salty component, save it for last. The longer the soup or vegetable cooks with the salt, the more chance it has to be driven into the food where it may have a negative health consequence and no flavor benefit. Similarly, when adding salt at the table, barely dusting it on the surface (a pinch has 150–250 mg sodium) and not stirring up the food too much will give a much more salty flavor for similar sodium levels. Again, you can get used to not adding it at all, but it will take time. The optimal approach is to leave added salt out.

You'll notice that we use a low-sodium tamari in many recipes because it imparts both salty and umami flavors. Be advised that manufacturers of soy sauce are aware of people's concern over excess sodium in their diets, and some label their products deceptively. One major brand lists its sodium content as 160 milligrams per serving. For comparison, the average soy sauce contains about 900 milligrams of sodium per tablespoon (500 mg for reduced-sodium varieties). So, how does a manufacturer make a soy sauce with 160 milligrams of sodium per serving? The serving size is ½ *teaspoon*! With an honest comparison, one finds it contains 960 milligrams of sodium per tablespoon—more than most other brands on the market. Tamari is an even thicker, less salty, Japanese version of soy sauce and typically doesn't use wheat, which gives it an edge for some people. The brand we use contains 490 milligrams of sodium per tablespoon and adds a wonderful umami punch.

Sugar

Sugar is the latest rage in food vilification. Everyone seems to be on the no-sugar train. We'll likely see a correction in glucophobia in the coming decade, but for now, sugar seems to have earned center-stage attention. This book has an entire section focused on sweets that aren't necessarily desserts. They are anytime meals. We explained why we've used molasses or maple syrup to sweeten things, and there are a host of nonsugar, manmade, and natural sweeteners that one can use. Like salt, sweet perception is highly adaptive and subject to habituation. Also like salt, some time away from excessively sweet foods made using artificial sweeteners or sugar will make the natural sweetness of fruits much more pronounced. It should be somewhat obvious that sugar—gram for gram—contained in a donut isn't metabolically equivalent to sugar obtained from a piece of fruit.

Flour

The closest thing we have in this book to baking a cake is falafel, and our use of flours is mostly limited to thickening sauces and gravies. Arrowroot is our go-to thickener in the kitchen. It gets a creamy thickness at a lower temperature than cornstarch and holds up better to acidic soups and sauces as often found in Asian cooking. We use cornstarch as well, but another good alternative is chickpea flour (gram flour). It can be used to batter vegetables like cauliflower for a deep-fried, breading-like texture. Our recipes use flours to thicken and add a creamy texture, and these three should provide enough flexibility to achieve this goal.

Our message here is simple. Don't let all the internet chatter on sugar, salt, and oil interfere with your ability to make a dish that contains a balance of sweet, salty, and fatty tastes. Likewise, having a

BASIC TASTE FOOD ADDITIVES IN OUR KITCHEN

- **Molasses:** adds a sweet but strong flavor that naturally limits using too much.
- **Nutritional yeast:** affectionately called "nooch," these yellow flakes add a funky, cheesy flavor, but it may be an acquired taste.
- **Low-sodium tamari:** our preferred method for adding salty flavor, as it also adds umami. We like Kikkoman Less Sodium Tamari.
- **Coconut aminos:** adds a salty flavor, but with a more neutral flavor than tamari.
- **Sodium-free seasoning:** adds flavor without salt. Our favorites include Mrs. Dash, Benson's Table Tasty, Daks, Kirkland No-Salt Seasoning, and Lawry's Salt-Free 17.
- **Hot sauces:** there are endless varieties from mild to super spicy, but watch the sodium content. We like Tabasco and Sriracha.
- **Cashews:** a neutral fat source for adding creamy texture to sauces and dressings.
- **Hempseeds:** a great one-to-one substitute for cashews for those with nut allergies.
- **Nondairy milks:** plain, unsweetened plant milks add creaminess. We keep shelf-stable varieties on hand as back-up.
- **Canned tomatoes and tomato paste:** provide a very consistent tomato flavor, and the paste is an excellent source of umami.
- **Lemon or lime juice and vinegars:** sour and tangy, these bring complexity and depth and can balance flavor when one might otherwise be tempted to add salt.
- **Anjinomoto Plus:** umami in a sprinkle. While not generally available in the United States, it is easily sourced internationally.

creamy, decadent texture is easy to achieve. When you substitute, think about hitting more than one taste at a time, such as adding tamari for both salty and umami flavors. This flavor duality is also true when using raw cashews to add both oleogustus with a creamy texture in sauces and dressings. Also, keep in mind that creating quality flavor might limit quantity and assist in bringing your daily eating into the dietary restriction range without any sense of deprivation.

WHAT SHOULD I EAT?

The answer is: vegetables, fruits, whole grains, legumes, mushrooms, nuts, seeds, herbs, and spices. That list, though....yes, we both love to say this list of ingredients over and over to our clients, audiences, and even for fun, to one another. This is what we want you to eat. It may sound a bit elementary, yet there is a profound body of evidence to support why these simple staples straight from the ground are all you need for sustainable success.

Vegetables and Fruits

If there is one thing all the major leading healthcare organizations agree on, it's the recommendation to eat more fruits and vegetables. The American Cancer Society recommends eating at least 2½ cups of fruits and vegetables daily to reduce cancer risk;[14] the American Heart Association suggests 4 to 5 servings of each per day for cardiovascular protection;[15] and the USDA suggests 2 cups of fruit and 2½ cups of vegetables in a 2,000-calorie-per-day diet.[16] Despite these recommendations, most everyone falls short on getting enough of these colorful, low-calorie, nutrient-dense, and health-promoting treasures.[17]

The World Health Organization (WHO) estimates that nearly 4 million deaths could be attributed to suboptimal fruit and vegetable consumption worldwide in 2017. Because there is ample evidence supporting the reduction in risk of noncommunicable (chronic) diseases with adequate consumption of these two crucial categories of food groups, the WHO recommends including 400 grams of vegetables and fruits per day to improve health and decrease disease risk.[18]

[19] (This does not include starchy vegetables.) Essentially, the classic endorsement for more fruits and veggies has merely garnered support with the ever-increasing volumes of new data.

Heading back to the Food Triangle, we separate out green leafy vegetables, cruciferous vegetables, mushrooms, stems, and bulbs at the top, as they are the most nutritionally-dense foods and they contain the fewest calories. Loaded with fiber, phytonutrients, and essential vitamins and minerals, they can be consumed in nearly unlimited quantities, and we encourage you to maximize your intake. Starchy vegetables and fruits live at the bottom, right side of the Food Triangle because, while still very high in similar key nutrients, these foods are denser in calories, also providing satiety and energy.

There are many ways to categorize vegetables and fruits—from botanical to nutritional and also culinary classifications—but the simplest way to consider nature's true power foods, is to:

1. **Aim to "eat the rainbow" and consume a wide variety of vibrant colors daily.** Some examples from the recipes ahead include red (strawberries, bell peppers, tomatoes, and red onion), orange (papaya, mango, sweet potato, and butternut squash), yellow (pineapple, lemon, sweet corn, and spaghetti squash), green (avocado, lime, asparagus, and broccoli), blue/purple (blueberries, plums, eggplant, and purple cabbage), and white (parsnips, cauliflower, onions, and jicama).

2. **Use the Food Triangle.** Emphasize top-triangle foods as the center of your meals. Include starchy vegetables and fruits more moderately and based on energy needs.

3. **Focus on fresh and frozen.** Prioritize fresh and frozen fruits and vegetables, either cooked or raw, over canned, jarred, or dried for optimal nutrition profiles.

Whole Grains

Grains, also referred to as cereals, are the edible seeds of grasses. They are considered "whole" when the germ, endosperm, and bran are intact, as opposed to when parts are refined through the milling process, which changes the structure and nutritional value. Although there aren't specific essential nutrients found in whole grains that can't be found in the other food categories, these foods have been staples throughout the world since recorded history began for several reasons. Not only are they low in cost, culinarily flexible, and satiating, but a diet high in whole grains has been associated with reduced risk of cardiovascular disease, type 2 diabetes, cancer, all-cause mortality, and mortality from respiratory disease, infectious disease, diabetes, and all noncardiovascular, non-cancer causes.[20] [21] [22]

Whole grains are from the grass family *Poaceae* and include barley, maize, millet, oats, rice, rye, teff, triticale, sorghum, wheat and its derivatives (e.g., emmer, farro, freekeh, and spelt), and wild rice. Amaranth, buckwheat, and quinoa are examples of pseudo-grains (or pseudo-cereals), which are nutritionally similar to the others, but from different botanical families.

Legumes

Legumes represent a broad category of seeds, pods, and other edible parts in the family of flowering plants known as *Leguminosae* or *Fabaceae*, and include beans, lentils, peas, and soyfoods (e.g., tofu and tempeh). Peanuts are also legumes, but nutritionally and culinarily, they are more similar to nuts and seeds.

Legumes are particularly noteworthy because of their extraordinary nutrition profile, health advantages, and diversity in the kitchen. As an exceptional source of slowly digestible fiber, including soluble and insoluble fibers and resistant starch, legumes help improve glycemic control, lower cholesterol, and enhance satiety. Legumes have a unique ability to fix nitrogen, making them rich sources of amino acids, including essential amino acids. They are high in indispensable minerals, such as iron, calcium, zinc, magnesium, phosphorus, potassium, and manganese, as well as B vitamins (especially folate), and phytonutrients, including isoflavones, lignans, lutein, and zeaxanthin.

One of the commonalities found amongst all of the Blue Zones (the longest lived populations across the world) is the regular consumption of legumes.[23] Associated with reduced risk for cardiovascular disease,[24] type 2 diabetes,[25] certain cancers,[26] and improved weight management,[27] [28] legumes play a key role in a healthspan-promoting diet.

Represented in this gem of a food group, and with examples sprinkled throughout the recipes in the chapters ahead, are an array of beans, peas, lentils, and soyfoods. They are nutritious and convenient cooked from scratch, from a can (preferably low- or no-sodium) or an aseptic package, or frozen. Enjoy them in soups, puréed into hummus or other spreads, tossed whole onto salads, blended in a sauce (especially white cannellini beans or silken tofu), or smashed into a burger patty (as in our Bean Burger Formulator, page 178).

Mushrooms

Though typically tossed into the vegetable category, mushrooms are technically fungi, providing unique culinary and nutritional features.[29] While there are more than 2,000 varieties of mushrooms that are edible, only a few are typically included in the Western diet, including button, crimini, portabella, shiitake, oyster, maitake, morel, and chanterelle.[30] [31] [32]

Used medicinally for thousands of years to promote health and longevity, mushroom consumption is associated with better nutrient intake and diet profile.[33] Mushrooms contain bioactive immune-enhancing

polysaccharides, essential amino acids, and minerals, including calcium, potassium, magnesium, iron, and zinc. When treated with UV light, irradiated mushrooms can be a good source of vitamin D2 (ergocalciferol).[34] Mushrooms provide vital health advantages, including antioxidant, cholesterol-lowering, antihypertensive, anti-inflammatory, liver protective, antidiabetic, antiviral, and antimicrobial properties, and also act as powerful prebiotics to positively impact the gut microbiome.[35] [36]

Culinarily speaking, fresh and dried mushrooms are a novel low-energy, low-sodium, and high-potassium source of umami. Their diverse textures can be used to substitute different types of meat and seafood. For example, finely minced portabella, oyster, crimini, or button mushrooms can replace ground meat; shredded king trumpet can replace pulled pork; sliced king oysters can be mock scallops; and lobster mushrooms can act as a stand-in for lobster. For added nutrition and umami flavor, sprinkle blended dried mushrooms (or Magic Mushroom Powder, page 242) over foods.

Nuts and Seeds

Nuts and seeds are foods that should be consumed regularly for health. Found at the bottom right of the food triangle, due to their energy density, they are exceptionally nutrient dense. Nuts and seeds offer a unique nutritional profile, including amino acids, such as L-arginine; monounsaturated and polyunsaturated fats (plus they are low in saturated fats); vitamins E, K, folate, and thiamine; essential minerals, especially calcium, copper, iron, magnesium, phosphorus, potassium, selenium, and zinc; and phytonutrients, such as phytosterols, lignans, and ellagic acid.

Nuts include tree nuts, which encompass almonds, Brazil nuts, cashews, hazelnuts, macadamias, pecans, pistachios, and walnuts, as well as legume seeds, such as peanuts. In the seeds category are chia, flax, hemp, poppy, pumpkin, sesame, and sunflower. Frequent consumption of nuts and seeds is associated with improved satiety, glucose control, cholesterol profiles, cognitive function, decreased mortality, and despite their high energy content, nut consumption helpfully influences weight management.[37] [38] [39] [40] [41]

Mixing up your intake with a variety of nuts and seeds is a good idea based on much of the research findings, and also because there are individual highlights throughout this food group. For example, Brazil nuts contain unusually hefty doses of selenium, an essential trace mineral that is a bit more challenging to find in other foods.[42] Interestingly, one clinical trial showed that a mere single serving (20 grams, approximately 4 Brazil nuts) was able to improve cholesterol profiles for an entire month.[43] Walnuts, chia seeds, flaxseeds, and hempseeds are loaded with heart-healthy omega-3 fatty acids. Almonds are part of the Portfolio diet, a special diet that also includes viscous fibers, plant sterols, and soyfoods, and has been shown to reduce cholesterol levels as powerfully as statins.[44] [45]

We recommend consuming one to two ounces of nuts and seeds daily. This category also includes nut and seed butters, two tablespoons of which count as an ounce. Because it is easy to overeat these foods—particularly by noshing on them hand-to-mouth when available—we advise using them as a base for sauces and dressings, as you will see demonstrated in the chapters ahead. An added perk of enjoying them this way, together with colorful fruits and vegetables, is that they enhance the absorption of the fat-soluble nutrients, such as carotenoids, also present in those foods.[46] [47] [48]

Herbs and Spices

Herbs and spices are the commonly grouped names of compounds given to the leaf, root, bark, berry, bud, seed, or stigma of a plant or flower used for the

THE 6 DAILY 3'S

Prioritize the most nutritionally important staples with the 6 Daily 3's. Aim to consume three servings each of green vegetables, other vegetables, fruits, nuts and seeds, and legumes. The sixth category is movement, as being physically active is also important on a daily basis.

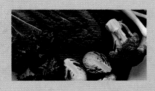

3 SERVINGS OF GREEN VEGETABLES
1 serving = 1 cup raw or ½ cup cooked
Examples include asparagus, bok choy, broccoli, cabbage, dandelion greens, kale, and any type of lettuce or sea vegetable.

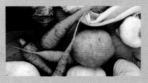

3 SERVINGS OF OTHER VEGETABLES
1 serving = 1 cup raw or ½ cup cooked
Aim to eat vegetables from the entire rainbow spectrum, such as cauliflower (white), beets (red), carrots (orange), corn (yellow), and egglant (purple).

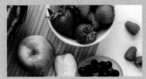

3 SERVINGS OF FRUIT
1 serving = 1 medium piece or 1 cup
Try to eat a variety of fruits, such as berries, grapes, mango, melon, pears, and plums.

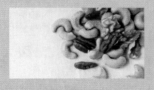

3 SERVINGS OF NUTS OR SEEDS
1 serving = 1 tablespoon seeds or ½ ounce nuts
Try almonds, cashews, walnuts, chia seeds, flaxseeds, hempseeds, and pumpkin seeds.

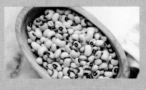

3 SERVINGS OF LEGUMES
1 serving = ½ cup
Examples include black beans, black-eyed peas, butter beans, chickpeas, kidney beans, lentils, and soyfoods such as tempeh and tofu.

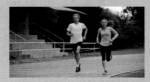

3 SERVINGS OF EXERCISE
1 serving = 20 minutes of activity
Exercise can be anything from light walking, stretching, and stair climbing to higher-intensity fitness bouts, such as weight lifting, jogging, and sports.

purpose of cooking, primarily to add or enhance flavor or color or for preservation. These ingredients also confer health benefits, including anti-inflammatory, antioxidant, antimicrobial, hypocholesterolemic, neuroprotective, antidiabetic, antiasthma, and anticarcinogenic effects, possibly due to their polyphenols (especially phenolic acids and flavonoids). Growing evidence suggests herbs and spices support gut health and protect against cardiovascular disease, neurodegenerative diseases, type 2 diabetes, and certain cancers.[49] [50]

From a flavor perspective, there is no limit to the diversity that can be invoked by the use of herbs and spices. For example, imagine a typical bowl of rice and beans. Known as a quintessential staple for nutritional balance and satiety in many places around the globe, this combination can be given a Mexican twist a la the Mexican Rice Burrito Bowl (page 155) with cumin, oregano, and chili powder. It could move in the direction of traditional Indian cooking using curry powder and garlic or in the style of traditional Louisiana red beans and rice with Cajun seasoning, thyme, sage, parsley, and cayenne pepper. Each of these recipes use similar base ingredients, but with vastly different flavor profiles.

Because of the vast medicinal properties and flavor-expansion potential, be sure to take advantage of herbs and spices throughout your meals and amp up the flavor with basil, cinnamon, cloves, coriander, cumin, fennel, fenugreek, ginger, mint, nutmeg, onion, oregano,

pepper, rosemary, sage, thyme, and turmeric. Although this may be intimidating for anyone not used to exploring the spice rack freely, use recipes (such as those in this book) to learn which flavors and combinations you prefer. As with anything, the practice of playing with herbs and spices will make it convenient, familiar, and enjoyable.

HOW TO USE THIS BOOK

We've attempted to design recipes that take shelf life into consideration and make efficient use of standard packaging sizes. For example, a can of beans typically contains 3½ servings of beans. Yet, who wants to put a half-serving of beans into a container and attempt to use it in a couple of days if you only need three servings? So, it's reasonable that we dump the whole can of beans into a recipe. Is serving an extra half-can of beans amongst two people a problem? Of course not, but now we need to increase the seasoning by a small amount, and so starts the rippling of the recipe causing a cascading juggle to balance the flavors. Food isn't packaged perfectly, and that's okay, but recognize that recipes aren't perfect, either, and there is always wiggle room for your personal adjustments and preferences. Unfortunately, this also means that your prior palate habits can easily move these recipes into a zone where you end up with the same diet you began with. Everything in diet is habit, and we are trying to help you move those habits into a more healthful direction.

For some of you, your salt intake has been adjusted nearly to zero and you might find some of these recipes too salty. Those of you who grab the salt shaker before you've even tasted the food might find the same recipe bland and unpalatable. Likewise, a similar argument can be made for sweet and oily. For this reason, we have included a range of oily, salty, sweet, sour, bitter, and umami flavors in our recipes, and this will serve as a foundational template for crafting your new healthspan habits. Increasing healthspan does not require that one eat perfectly, but "rare and appropriate" has no meaning when decadent food choices are frequent and over the top.

If you have adapted to a no-salt-added lifestyle, you should immediately recognize the ingredients in our recipes that need to be adjusted. We have tried to keep them within a sweet spot such that people new to this lifestyle can succeed as well as people who are already savvy to eating to the right of the Food Triangle. We can only imagine the debates that will ensue over calling for a teaspoon of sesame oil or not specifying "no salt added" tomatoes. But for the vast majority of people eating this way for the first time, there will be a period of adjustment. We should recognize that the culinary norms throughout the world provide ample evidence that the most pleasure in food occurs in a palate balance that doesn't necessarily fit healthspan patterns. Restaurants and fast-food chains aren't wrong for serving what they serve. Health is your business; their business is selling food. They sell what we think tastes good. At the same time, success is predicated on avoiding using perfect as a barrier to progress. In short, get as close to 100 percent of the days 90 percent plus correct, and don't plan on "cheat days."

Comfort food

Some people will make choices based on food volume; for others, it may be a love of sweets. Some like savory or spicy; others can't get enough umami or salt. No matter what your acquired food drive is, be it stuffing your belly or chasing the perfect bite of a decadent delicacy, your food habits can be changed at any age.

One of the biggest problems in changing your diet is that the word "diet" is synonymous with weight loss. Sustaining a caloric deficit and eating for healthspan and weight maintenance are two completely unrelated goals and physiologies. Conflating these two important diet definitions is probably why success in either pursuit is fleeting. If you have some weight to lose, it's probably best that you table that goal for now and dedicate three to six months of no deviation from the eating patterns described in this book. Many begin to lose weight without trying, and once your palate adapts to the flavor and variety described in this book, you can eat a shockingly large volume of food and not gain weight.

Of course, our goal here is not a contest to see how much food you can stuff in your belly and maintain weight. The innumerable birthdays, anniversaries, retirements, holidays, and, yes, even wakes and funerals too often seem like team food-swallowing contests. When faced with celebration junk food, it's probably better that you chow down on an entire recipe (perhaps even doubling it) in this book than participating in said team-swallowing celebrations as a *de facto* "rare and appropriate." It might be the time for deviation, but it also might not. These events occur so often that everyone will need to pick and choose them carefully. Like we discussed with picking the perfect lunch spot, making this decision alone, especially during a time of lifestyle transition, will always be the easiest and most successful route.

Cooking for Others

If you are responsible for preparing meals for friends and immediate family, it's more practical to fix them what they want and serve one or more of these recipes alongside that than it is to have them read this book before they show up to the dinner table. Your diet doesn't need to be their diet. Since the people you'll be preparing food for are already comfortable with soups, salads, sides, and sweets, the only difference between these recipes and what they already like mostly distills down to how sweet, salty, and oily the recipe is. Providing them a comfortable way to adjust sweet, salty, and oily to their palate preferences is a far

more productive way of opening a dialogue about why, what, and how you eat than attacking and criticizing their food habits or cultural norms. After all, it's not a coincidence that salt, pepper, MSG, vinegar, oil, and hot sauce, along with hosts of other culturally significant condiments, are available on tables around the world.

If you want to set an example for your children or partner, saying as little as you can and just eating your meals herein will be far more persuasive than telling them how unhealthy their eating habits have become. In general, people make food choices far more often based on emulation than logic or reason. Think about the messages you are inadvertently sending when you tell a child, "Finish your healthy vegetables and then you can have a decadent dessert;" "Okay, I'll take just one bite, but I'm on a diet;" or "I used to love eating that before my diet changed." The implicit message is that you are depriving yourself of food pleasure for no obvious or immediate gain. Unless you develop a food habit for acutely toxic substances—like certain mushrooms and hemlock tea—what you eat today and its connection to health benefit or demise is likely separated by decades. Making the emotional choice in the moment is always far easier than suppressing the hedonistic pleasure and making a long-term rational choice. What we have found working with

"Your diet doesn't need to be their diet."

hundreds of clients is that it's far easier to move what we find pleasurable today than to suppress and deprive over months, years, and decades. You can't cognitively inhibit a biological urge forever. Eventually, the urge wins. But you can modify the urge. We call this the "new normal," and the recipes you'll find on these pages provide a rapid healthspan solution to permanent lifestyle transformation.

Final Thoughts

We believe food is a fundamental part of our social interaction with others. Yet, it's also the primary change that you can make to reduce or eliminate many avoidable chronic diseases. We realize it takes a while for the new normal to take hold and to find your new favorite food, but we have seen this success directly in hundreds of clients and indirectly in thousands on our social media streams. We broke a lot of cookbook rules so you could have a solid foundation for the science behind our recommendations. We hope you can use the following recipes to develop those new habits and ultimately protect against "rare and appropriate" becoming "frequent and inappropriate."

If you have weight issues or other nutritionally induced chronic diseases, it will take some effort, but the recipes are some of the same we've used to have profound impact on people. Ultimately, there are so many unhealthful food

choices we repeat, and those never seem to feel limiting and boring. If you can just replace those with 8 to 10 recipes or menu items inspired by the new favorite foods found in this book, we know you will be successful. We're excited to be part of your new healthspan-centered life.

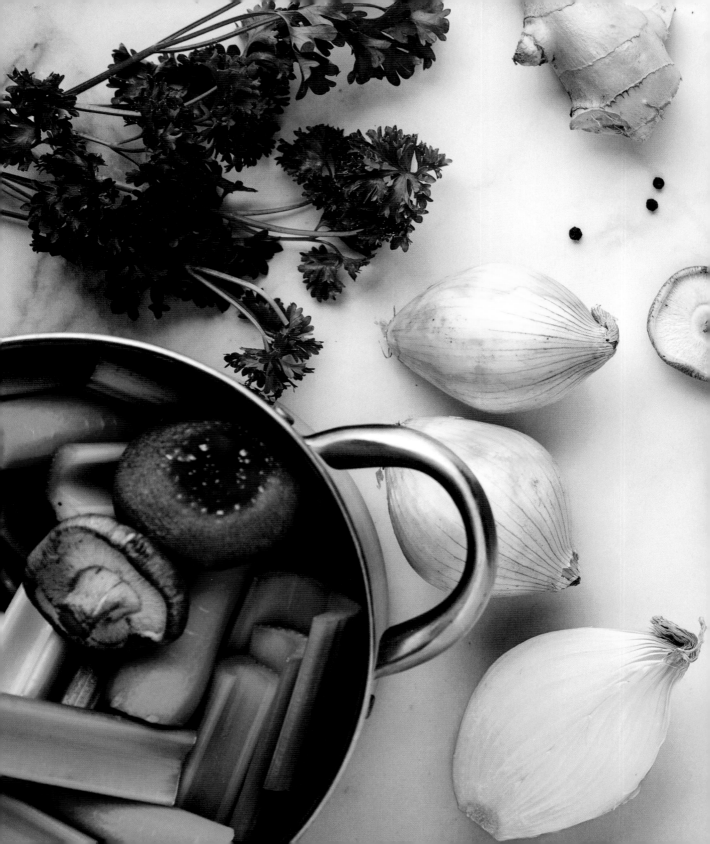

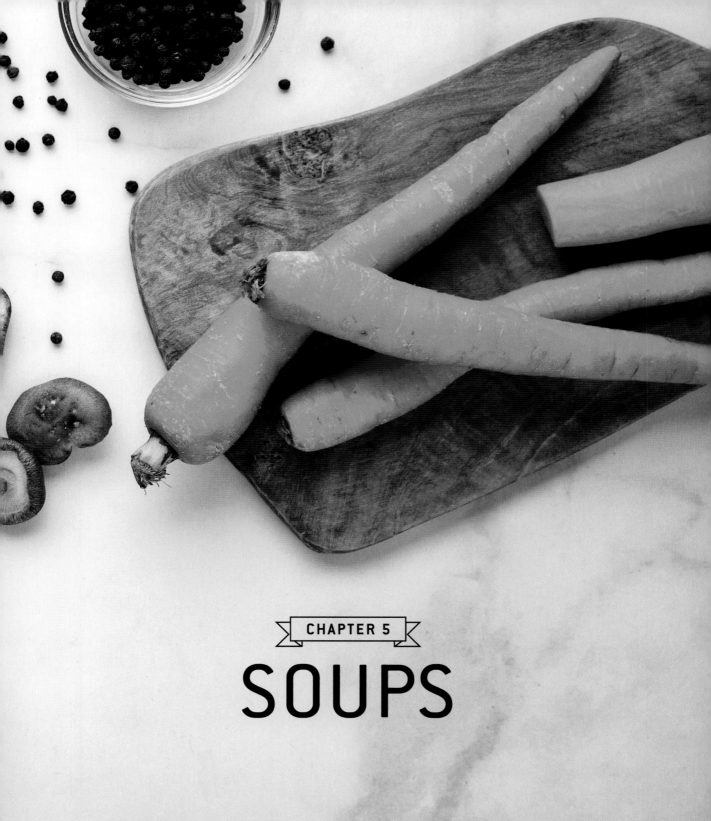

CHAPTER 5

SOUPS

SIMPLE STOCK

PREP TIME: **15 MINUTES**
COOK TIME: **1 HOUR 10 MINUTES**
YIELD: **2 QUARTS**

INGREDIENTS

4 cups roughly chopped yellow onion (about 4 onions)

2 cups roughly chopped carrots (about 4 carrots)

2 cups roughly chopped celery (about 4 stalks)

½ cup sliced shiitake mushrooms

3 bay leaves

1 tsp black peppercorns

On the shelves of most grocery stores across the United States are dozens of stocks and broths made from chicken, beef, "bones," more chicken, more beef, and more "bones." Often, there are one or two vegetable options, but it is more challenging to find low-sodium vegetable broth or low-sodium no-chicken broth (one of our favorites). Making your own homemade version is a simple solution to save money, completely control ingredients, and enhance flavor.

STOVETOP DIRECTIONS

1   In a large stock pot, dry sauté the onions for 3 to 4 minutes until golden and translucent, adding a spash of water if needed to prevent burning. Add the carrots, celery, mushrooms, bay leaves, peppercorns, and 10 cups water.

2   Bring to a boil and cook covered for 15 minutes. Reduce the heat, and simmer covered for about 35 minutes. Add water as needed to keep the vegetables covered.

3   Strain the stock into a large bowl, squeezing as much liquid as possible from the vegetables. Discard the solids. Transfer the stock from the bowl to quart-size glass Mason jars for storage. Store in the refrigerator for up to 1 week or in the freezer for 4 to 6 months.

MULTI-COOKER DIRECTIONS

1   Using the SAUTE function, dry sauté the onions until translucent, adding a splash of water to prevent them from burning.

2   Add the carrots, celery, bay leaves, mushrooms, peppercorns, and 10 cups water. Set the PRESSURE function for 40 minutes. Allow the pressure to naturally release for 10 minutes and then manually release.

3   Strain the stock into a large bowl, squeezing as much liquid as possible from the vegetables. Discard the solids. Transfer the stock from the bowl to quart-size glass Mason jars for storage. Store in the refrigerator for up to 1 week or in the freezer for 4 to 6 months.

✎   **NOTES:** This stock is neutral in flavor, making it a good base for many recipes. Consider adding any of the following for a stronger flavor:

+ 1 bunch scallions
+ 5–6 sprigs flat-leaf (Italian) parsley
+ 5–6 sprigs fresh thyme
+ 3–4 Swiss chard leaves

To make Suppengrün (German soup base), use celeriac (celery root) in place of celery stalks and leeks in place of yellow onion.

DASHI

PREP TIME: **5 MINUTES**
COOK TIME: **20 MINUTES**
YIELD: **1 QUART**

INGREDIENTS

¼ cup dried shiitake mushrooms, sliced

1 tsp nori flakes

2- to 3-in strip kombu

Dashi is a Japanese soup stock, traditionally made with sea vegetables, dried fish (usually bonito flakes), and dried mushrooms. It is used for miso soup, noodle dishes, and stews. Although there are only a few ingredients, this plant-based combination sets the stage for a savory, umami, flavor-filled base.

1   In a saucepan, combine mushrooms and 4 cups water and bring to a boil over high heat. Once boiling, reduce heat to low. Add the nori and kombu and allow to steep for 15 to 20 minutes. Water should be hot but not simmering; if heated too vigorously, the kombu can get slimy.

2   Strain the liquid into a bowl, squeezing as much liquid as possible from the solids. Discard the solids. Transfer the dashi from the bowl to a quart-size glass Mason jar for storage. Store in the refrigerator for up to 1 week or in the freezer for 4 to 6 months.

GARLICKY GINGER "ZOODLES"
with Mushrooms and Red Cabbage

PREP TIME: **10 MINUTES**
COOK TIME: **15 MINUTES**
YIELD: **5 CUPS**

INGREDIENTS

¼ cup dried wood ear mushrooms

4 tsp white miso paste

2 tbsp warm water

1 tbsp minced fresh ginger

1 bunch scallions, chopped (reserve green parts for garnish)

2 tsp sesame oil

2–3 garlic cloves, minced

4 cups **Dashi** (page 97) or low-sodium vegetable broth

3–4 slices daikon radish, sliced round and then halved

1 tsp nori flakes

¼ cup sliced shiitake mushrooms

2 cups spiralized zucchini ("zoodles")

2 cups shredded red cabbage (slice in long, thin shreds)

1 tbsp low-sodium tamari

Optional garnishes

Toasted sesame seeds

Ichimi togarashi (Japanese ground red chili pepper)

Shichimi togarashi or nanami togarashi (Japanese spice blends)

Wood ear mushrooms have a wonderful texture and flavor, a history of medicinal use, and the look of actual ears. The dried versions expand a surprising amount when soaked in water and thus, they are a key ingredient in this fun, lighter udon soup loaded with fresh vegetables.

1 Place the wood ear mushrooms in a small bowl, add about 2 cups water, and set aside, allowing them to rehydrate. In a separate small bowl, combine the miso paste and 2 tablespoons warm water, stir, and set aside to dissolve.

2 In a large saucepan, dry sauté the ginger and the white part of the scallions until softened and fragrant. Add just enough water or broth to prevent them from completely drying out. Push the ginger and scallions to the edge of the pan and drizzle sesame oil into the center of the pan. Add the garlic to the small puddle of oil and sauté for 30 to 60 seconds, or until golden, being careful not to scorch. Toss to combine ingredients.

3 Add the vegetable broth, radishes, nori flakes, and both the shiitake and rehydrated wood ear mushrooms. Bring to a boil and then reduce heat. Cover and simmer for 5 minutes. (See note on noodles if using dry ramen, udon, or soba. Add those here and allow to cook, per instructions.)

4 If using zoodles, add them along with the cabbage, and simmer 4 to 5 minutes, until softened. Stir in the dissolved miso paste and tamari and remove from heat.

5 Divide evenly between two bowls to serve, making sure each bowl gets an equal amount of zoodles, radishes, mushrooms, scallions, cabbage, and broth. Garnish with sliced scallions, toasted sesame seeds, and seasonings, as desired.

NOTES: This dish can be made with ramen, udon, or soba noodles, but these should be reserved for the rare special occasion. Many grocery stores sell zucchini spirals (or "zoodles") in the prepared food section, which is a bonus for convenience.

If wood ear mushrooms are unavailable, substitute shiitake mushrooms.

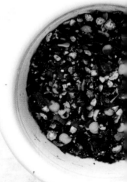

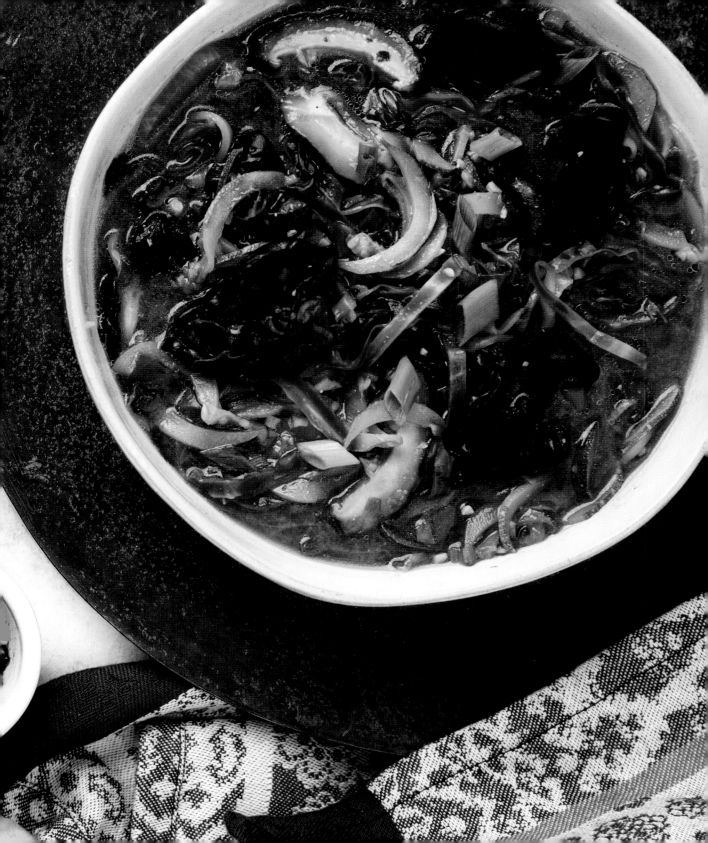

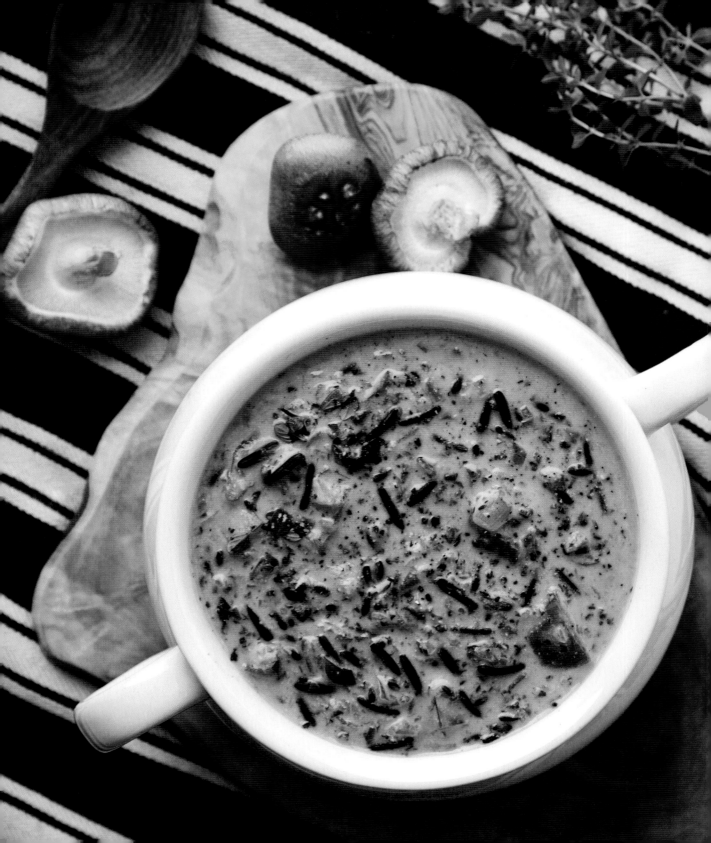

MUSHROOM WILD RICE BISQUE

PREP TIME: **15 MINUTES**
COOK TIME: **55 MINUTES**
YIELD: **5 CUPS**

INGREDIENTS

½ cup uncooked wild rice, rinsed

½ cup raw cashews

2 tsp arrowroot powder

⅔ cup unsweetened nondairy milk

1 cup diced yellow onion

1 cup diced celery

4oz fresh gourmet mushroom blend (or baby bella, brown, and/or oyster), sliced

3 garlic cloves, minced

¼ cup white wine

3 cups **Simple Stock** (page 96) or low-sodium vegetable broth

1 tbsp fresh thyme leaves, plus more to garnish

2 tbsp nutritional yeast

1 tbsp low-sodium tamari

2 tsp anchovy-free Worcestershire sauce

1 tbsp freshly squeezed lemon juice

Freshly ground black pepper, to taste

Sipping up this cozy bisque feels like being wrapped in a warm blanket in front of the fireplace. Comforting and creamy, hearty and satisfying, these simple flavors are decadent. Take it up a notch with a crusty roll and a glass of wine (some for the soup, plus some for the chef) and you will feel pampered.

1 Prepare the wild rice. In a medium saucepan, bring 1½ cups water to a boil. Once boiling, add the rice, reduce heat to low, cover, and simmer for 55 minutes, or according to package instructions.

2 Meanwhile, in a blender, combine the cashews and arrowroot powder. Pulse until a fine powder forms, but not enough to create a paste. Scrape the corners of the blender with a small spatula to make sure all the powder is free. Add the nondairy milk and blend until fully combined and creamy. Set aside.

3 Heat a large saucepan over medium-high heat. Dry sauté the onions and celery with 1 to 2 tablespoons water—enough to avoid burning while still allowing browning on the bottom of the pan—until onions are translucent. Add the mushrooms and a small amount of additional water (1–2 tbsp) to allow mushrooms to release their liquid. Once liquid is released, push vegetables to the periphery and add the minced garlic to the center of the pan. Sauté the garlic for 30 to 60 seconds

4 Deglaze the pan with the wine, stirring to combine all ingredients, and scraping any brown bits off the bottom of the pan. Stir in the broth and bring to a boil. Reduce the heat to low and simmer for 7 to 8 minutes. Stir in the cashew cream and simmer until the bisque thickens, 3 to 5 minutes.

5 Add the thyme, nutritional yeast, tamari, and Worcestershire sauce. Stir to combine. Add the lemon juice, 1 teaspoon at a time, tasting as you go, and adjust according to taste.

6 Using an immersion blender, pulse the soup 2 to 3 times to thicken and blend flavors, but do not purée. Add the cooked wild rice and stir to combine. Garnish with thyme and serve hot with a sprinkle of black pepper.

✎ **NOTE:** For the most efficient use of time, begin cooking the rice and then prepare the remaining ingredients.

EASY PEASY SPLIT PEA LENTIL SOUP

PREP TIME: **5 MINUTES**
COOK TIME: **60 MINUTES**
YIELD: **7 CUPS**

INGREDIENTS

8 cups **Simple Stock** (page 96) or low-sodium vegetable broth

3 bay leaves

½ cup dried shiitake mushrooms, crumbled

1½ cups dried split peas, rinsed

1½ cups dried red lentils, rinsed

1 tbsp fresh thyme, stems removed

½ tsp onion powder

½ tsp garlic powder

1 tsp smoked paprika

Liquid smoke, to taste

Freshly ground black pepper, to taste

Freshly squeezed lemon juice, to taste

Available throughout the year and exceptionally shelf stable, both split peas and lentils are perfect dry staples to keep stocked for quick, nutritious, and delicious meals. Because we delved into the superior nutrition and myriad health advantages of consuming legumes in Chapter 4, here is just one of the many easy ways to delight in your daily dose of this key food group.

1 Heat a large saucepan or Dutch oven over medium-high heat. Once hot, add the vegetable broth, bay leaves, and shiitake mushrooms, and bring to a boil. Once boiling, add the split peas and lentils. Reduce heat to low and cover partially. Simmer for 50 to 60 minutes, stirring occasionally, until the lentils and split peas have broken down to your desired texture.

2 Add the thyme, onion powder, garlic powder, and paprika, and simmer for an additional 5 minutes to allow the flavors to come together. Taste and add a dash of liquid smoke, a sprinkle of black pepper, and a squeeze of lemon, as needed. Remove the bay leaves and serve hot.

FIESTA CORN STEW

PREP TIME: **10 MINUTES**
COOK TIME: **45 MINUTES**
YIELD: **12 CUPS**

INGREDIENTS

2 cups corn kernels, fresh or frozen

1 cup chopped white onion

1 cup chopped celery

1 cup chopped green bell pepper

6 garlic cloves, thinly sliced

1 (15oz) can black beans, liquid reserved

1 (15oz) can pinto beans, drained and rinsed

1 (28oz) can low-sodium diced tomatoes

1 (6oz) can tomato paste (optional for more robust tomato flavor)

2 cups cubed butternut squash

1 tbsp chili powder

1 tsp chipotle powder

1 tsp dried Mexican oregano

1 tsp smoked paprika

4 cups **Simple Stock** (page 96) or low-sodium vegetable broth

¼ cup fresh cilantro leaves, stems removed (optional)

¼ cup pickled jalapeños, rinsed (optional)

To serve

Lime wedges

Warmed corn tortillas, cut into quarters

Pinch of cayenne

This is a fiesta in a bowl! Sweet roasted corn and butternut squash meets tangy simmering tomatoes and warm spicy flavors of Mexico. We love to make this recipe in huge batches (as evidenced by its large yield), so we can enjoy some right away and freeze leftovers in individual containers for future fiestas.

1 In a medium nonstick pan, toast the corn over high heat, stirring occasionally, for 10 to 20 minutes or until it begins to brown. Set aside.

2 Heat a large saucepan over medium-high heat. Once hot, add the onions, celery, and bell pepper and dry sauté until the onions are translucent. Add 1 to 2 tablespoons water or broth—just enough to keep the pan from completely drying out. Add the garlic and sauté for 60 to 90 seconds, being careful to brown but not burn.

3 Add the black beans (with liquid), pinto beans, diced tomatoes, tomato paste (if using), butternut squash, chili powder, chipotle powder, Mexican oregano, smoked paprika, and broth. Stir to combine and bring to a boil. Reduce the heat and simmer on low for 25 to 30 minutes, or until the squash is tender.

4 Stir in the roasted corn and optional cilantro and jalapeños and simmer for 5 minutes more. Serve hot with lime wedges, warmed corn tortillas, and a pinch of cayenne, as desired for added heat.

HOT AND SOUR SHIITAKE UDON

PREP TIME: **30 MINUTES**
COOK TIME: **20 MINUTES**
YIELD: **10 CUPS**

INGREDIENTS

1 bundle (90g) udon noodles

1 tbsp minced ginger

2 bunches scallions, sliced (reserve 2 tbsp of green portion for garnish)

1lb shiitake mushrooms, stems removed and tops sliced

1 tsp sesame oil

1 tbsp minced garlic

6 cups **Dashi** (page 97) or low-sodium vegetable broth

2 tbsp low-sodium tamari

¼ cup freshly squeezed lemon juice

2 tbsp seasoned rice vinegar

15oz firm tofu, cut into ½-in cubes

½ cup shredded red cabbage

½ cup shredded green cabbage

1 cup shredded carrots

Freshly ground black pepper or shichimi togarashi (Japanese seven spice blend), to taste

Fancy restaurants call this Asian Fusion. We call it comfort food. Fortifying this hot and sour broth with tofu, shiitake mushrooms, and ample colorful veggies makes this a satisfying winner year-round—and that's before we mention udon noodles! It's flavor, culture, and nutrition all in one colorful bowl.

1. Cook the udon noodles according to package directions, rinse with cold water, and set aside.

2. Heat a large stockpot over medium-high heat. Once hot, sauté the ginger and scallions with 1 to 2 tablespoons water until aromatic, 1 to 2 minutes. Add the shiitake mushrooms and another tablespoon of water and sauté until softened, 2 to 5 minutes.

3. Push the ingredients to the side of the pot and drizzle the sesame oil in the center. Add garlic to the small puddle of oil and sauté for 30 to 60 seconds or until golden, being careful not to scorch. Stir to combine all ingredients.

4. Add the vegetable broth and tamari and bring to a boil. Once boiling, reduce heat to low, cover, and simmer for 5 minutes. Add the lemon juice, rice vinegar, tofu, cabbage, and carrots, and simmer for 2 minutes more to heat the tofu through and soften the vegetables. Season with black pepper or shichimi togarashi to taste.

5. To each bowl, add your desired portion of udon noodles and ladle the broth, tofu, and vegetables over top. Garnish with reserved scallion greens and enjoy immediately.

NOTE: You can simplify shopping by using either red or green cabbage, but use approximately 1 cup total.

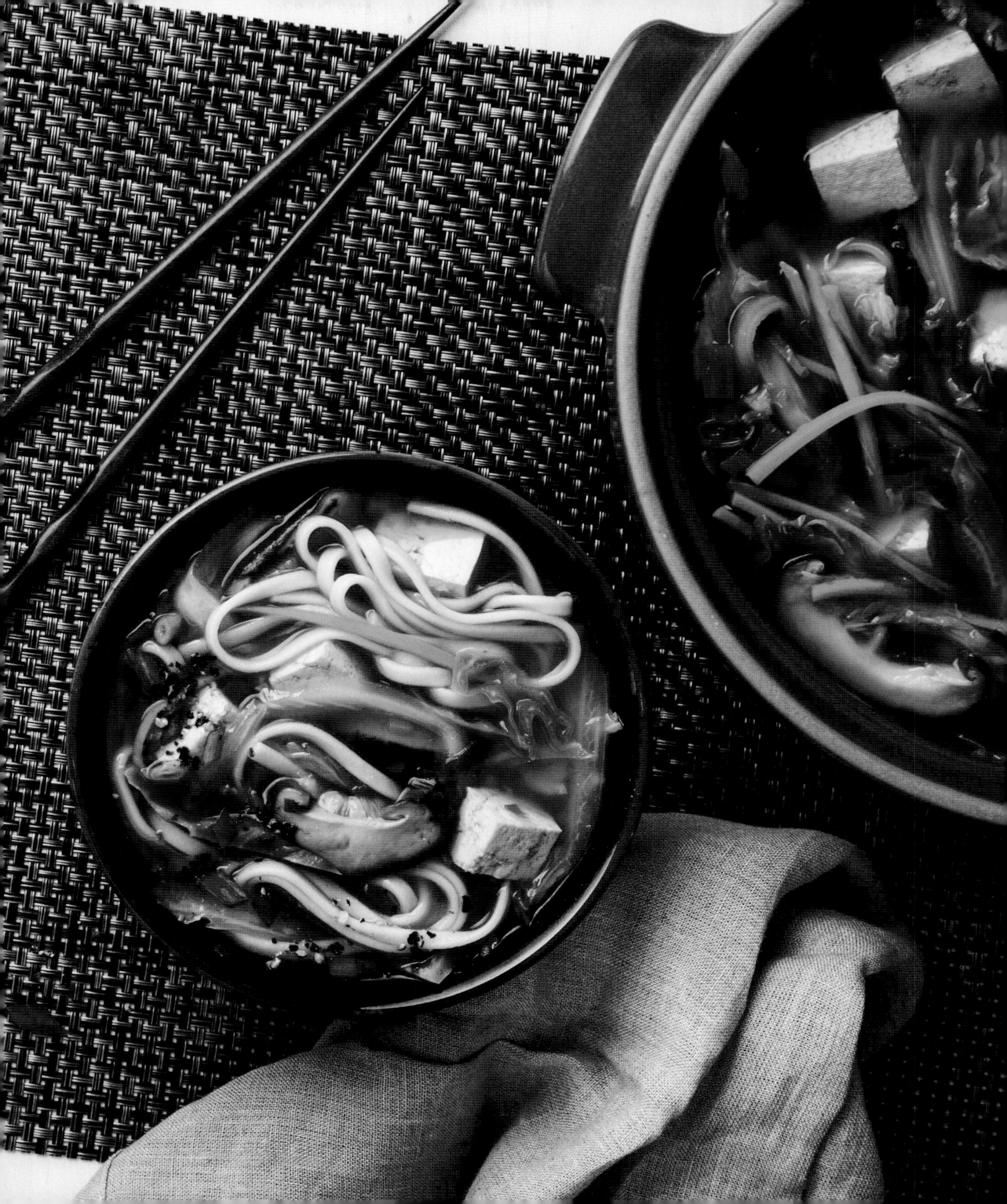

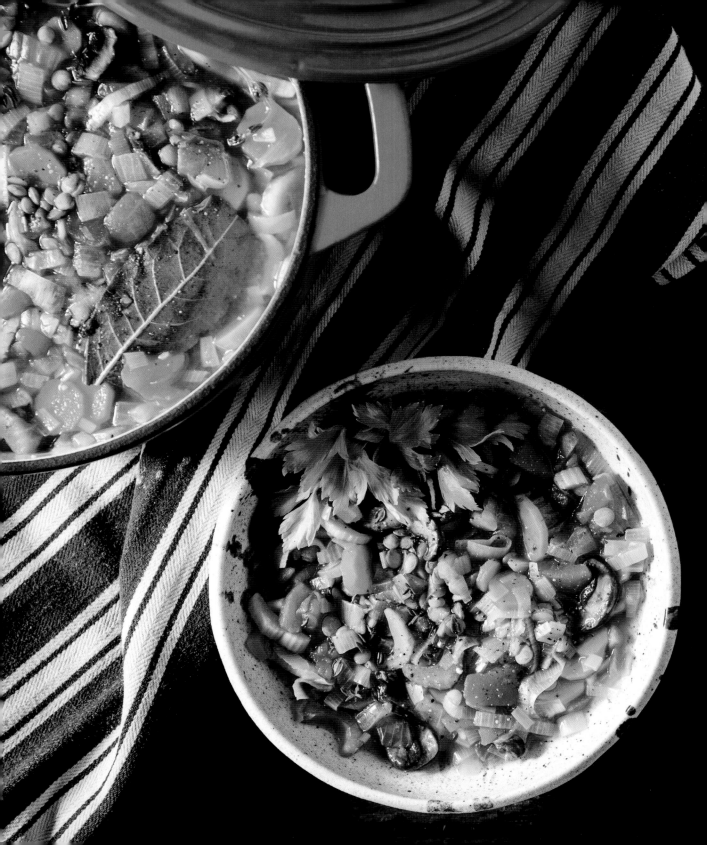

RUSTIC FRENCH LENTIL SOUP

PREP TIME: **15 MINUTES**
COOK TIME: **45 MINUTES**
YIELD: **8 CUPS**

INGREDIENTS

2 cups chopped yellow onions

2 cups thinly sliced leeks

1 cup sliced baby bella mushrooms

1 cup thinly sliced celery (reserve leaves for garnish)

1 cup thinly sliced carrots

2 garlic cloves, minced

6 cups **Simple Stock** (page 96) or low-sodium vegetable broth

1 bay leaf

½ tsp ground cumin

1 tbsp fresh thyme leaves

½ tsp freshly ground black pepper

1 (15oz) can diced tomatoes

1 tsp low-sodium tamari

1 cup dried Le Puy lentils (French green lentils), picked over and rinsed

¼ cup red wine or 2 tbsp red wine vinegar

Cashew Parmesan Sprinkle (optional, page 239), to serve

Celery leaves or parsley, chopped, to garnish

Le Puy lentils, known as "Lentilles Vertes du Puy," are small, dense, and flavorful green lentils, originally produced in Le Puy-en-Velay, in the Auvergne region of France. Known as a "poor man's caviar," this hearty lentil nutritiously replaces meat in this classic, comforting, and satisfying soup.

1 Heat a large stockpot over medium-high heat. Dry sauté the onions and leeks with as little water as possible for 3 to 4 minutes or until they begin to soften. Add the mushrooms and continue to sauté for 5 to 6 minutes until they release the water and the onions and leeks begin to brown.

2 Add the celery and carrots and sauté for 5 minutes more. Add the garlic and sauté for 30 to 60 seconds until browned, taking care not to scorch.

3 Add the broth and stir, scraping any browned bits from the bottom of the pan. Add the bay leaf, cumin, thyme, black pepper, tomatoes, tamari, and lentils. Bring to a boil, reduce heat, and simmer for 20 to 25 minutes until the lentils are tender. If too much liquid evaporates, you can add a little water to keep the lentils and vegetables covered.

4 Remove from heat and stir in the red wine. Serve with grated Cashew Parmesan Sprinkle, if desired, and garnish with celery leaves or parsley. Serve hot.

WEST AFRICAN GROUNDNUT STEW

PREP TIME: **15 MINUTES**
COOK TIME: **30 MINUTES**
YIELD: **4 SERVINGS**

INGREDIENTS

2 cups chopped yellow onion

1 sweet potato, peeled and cut into ½-in cubes

1 cup chopped green bell pepper

2 cups **Simple Stock** (page 96) or low-sodium vegetable broth, divided

4 cups chopped eggplant

1 cup chopped red cabbage

1 cup sliced okra, fresh or frozen

1 garlic clove, minced

1 (15oz) can low- or no-sodium diced tomatoes

¼ cup creamy peanut butter (see note)

1 tbsp ground hempseeds

¼–½ tsp cayenne, to taste

1 tsp freshly ground black pepper

This recipe is based on a classic West African stew, which is often made with meat and served with a starchy side, such as rice, plantains, or potatoes. In this version, we add the starch directly to the dish for a hearty, satisfying, one-pot meal. Traditionally, it is often made with scotch bonnet peppers, which are extraordinarily hot. If you like the heat, you can bump up the cayenne or even scout out a scotch bonnet (a close cousin of the habanero).

1   Heat a large saucepan or Dutch oven over medium-high heat. Once hot, add the onions and sauté with about 1 tablespoon water—use enough to avoid burning while still allowing browning on the bottom of the pan—for 5 minutes or until the onions are translucent.

2   Add the sweet potato, bell pepper, and ¼ cup broth. Sauté for 5 minutes, until the vegetables begin to soften. Stir in the eggplant, cabbage, okra, and garlic. Cover and simmer for 5 more minutes. Stir in the tomatoes and simmer for 3 to 5 minutes more.

3   While the vegetables cook, in a bowl or blender, combine the remaining 1¾ cups broth, peanut butter, and ground hempseeds, stirring or blending until smooth. Add the broth mixture to the stew and season with cayenne and black pepper to taste.

4   Simmer 15 to 20 minutes, or until all vegetables are tender. Serve hot.

✎ **NOTE:** You can substitute ½ cup fresh roasted peanuts for the peanut butter. Spread ½ cup peanuts on a baking sheet and roast at 350°F for 15 minutes. Toss the peanuts on the pan and roast 3 to 5 more minutes. They will continue cooking after you remove them from the oven. If using peanuts instead of peanut butter, add 1 tablespoon low-sodium tamari or a pinch of salt to the stew at the end of cooking to replace the salt that is typically found in peanut butter.

CRABBY CHEF FREEZER SOUP

PREP TIME: **5 MINUTES**
COOK TIME: **25 MINUTES**
YIELD: **4 SERVINGS**

INGREDIENTS

1 medium onion, diced

1lb (3 cups) frozen mixed
   vegetables, such as succotash

15oz frozen okra

15oz frozen cauliflower

1 (28oz) can crushed fire-roasted
   tomatoes

4 cups **Simple Stock** (page 96) or
   low-sodium vegetable broth

3 bay leaves

1 tsp celery seeds

4 tsp low-sodium Old Bay Seasoning

3 tbsp apple cider vinegar

½ tsp smoked paprika

¼ tsp cayenne pepper

Growing up in Maryland, on the banks of the Chesapeake Bay, Ray slurped down bowls of "she crab" soup. We both love Old Bay Seasoning, but it can be high in sodium. We used a low-sodium version in this recipe and added pounds of colorful vegetables. You'll gobble it up (gracefully, of course). This is an easy, fast soup to make for those days when you're feeling too crabby to cook. It uses freezer and pantry staples, which are perfect for last-minute meals, including frozen vegetable blends, canned tomatoes, and seasonings. And when it's finished cooking, you can put it back in the freezer for an even faster meal next time.

1   Heat a large saucepan or Dutch oven over medium-high heat. Once hot, dry sauté the onions for 3 to 4 minutes until they begin to brown.

2   Add the frozen mixed vegetables, frozen okra, frozen cauliflower, crushed tomatoes, vegetable broth, bay leaves, celery seeds, Old Bay Seasoning, apple cider vinegar, smoked paprika, and cayenne pepper. Cover and bring to a boil.

3   Once boiling, remove the lid, reduce heat to low, and simmer for 20 minutes. Adjust the seasoning as needed, and serve hot.

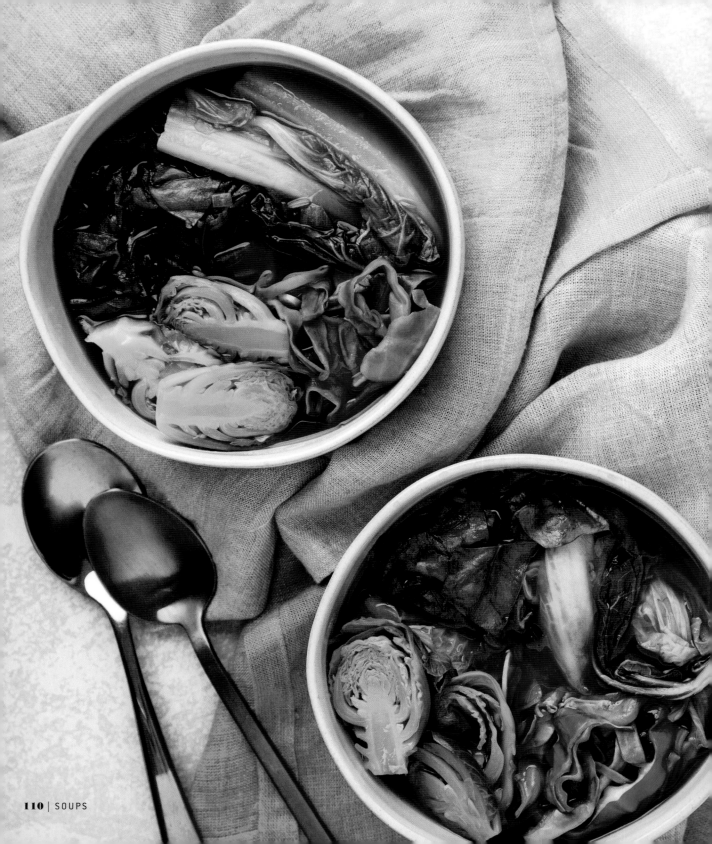

Hearty Cruciferous
CABBAGE STEW

PREP TIME: **15 MINUTES**
COOK TIME: **30 MINUTES**
YIELD: **8 CUPS**

INGREDIENTS

1 small yellow onion, diced

2 small parsnips, cut into thick slices

1 cup Brussels sprouts, sliced lengthwise in thirds

4 garlic cloves, sliced

2 cups unpeeled, cubed golden potatoes

4 cups **Simple Stock** (page 96) or low-sodium vegetable broth

1 (15oz) can diced tomatoes

1 tbsp caraway seeds (more or less to taste)

¼ cup apple cider vinegar

1 tbsp molasses

1 tbsp low-sodium tamari

1 cup chopped napa cabbage

1 cup chopped red cabbage

1 cup chopped Swiss chard, thick stems removed

4–5 baby bok choy, quartered

Freshly ground black pepper, to taste

Perhaps this is better titled, "Top Triangle Soup," as it is loaded with those crucial cruciferous vegetables highlighted at the top of the Food Triangle. Chock-full of glucosinolates and bright phytonutrient color, this is a hearty, vibrant cabbage stew. We wanted to create our take on a simple recipe that has fueled families in austere times. Too often, we tend to be steeped in culinary excess. The irony is that fresh, delicious, and nutritious plant-sourced food is now considered a luxury and is available ubiquitously and year-round.

1   Heat a large saucepan or Dutch oven over medium-high heat. Once hot, sauté the onions, parsnips, and Brussels sprouts with as little water as possible—use just enough to avoid burning—until the onions are translucent and begin to caramelize.

2   Add the garlic and cook for 30 to 45 seconds, until golden brown, taking care not to burn. Add the potatoes and broth and bring to a boil. Simmer for 15 minutes until the potatoes begin to soften but aren't quite fully cooked. (They will cook further as the vegetables steam.)

3   Add the tomatoes, caraway seeds, apple cider vinegar, molasses, and tamari. Simmer for 1 to 2 minutes to meld the flavors, and then taste and add more vinegar, molasses, or tamari as needed.

4   Add the napa cabbage, red cabbage, Swiss chard, and bok choy, allowing it all to float on top. Cover to steam for about 5 minutes, until the desired tenderness is reached.

5   Ladle out the vegetables from the top of the pot and add an equal portion to each bowl, or stir everything together before serving. This soup is even better— although not quite as colorful—the second day.

CHANA MASALA

PREP TIME: **10 MINUTES**
COOK TIME: **25 MINUTES**
YIELD: **6 CUPS**

INGREDIENTS

2 cups diced yellow onion

1 fresh hot pepper, such as serrano, jalapeño, or red chile, cut into rounds

2 tsp minced garlic

2 tsp minced fresh ginger

1 (28oz) can fire-roasted diced tomatoes

2 (15oz) cans low-sodium chickpeas, drained and rinsed, or 3 cups cooked chickpeas

1 tbsp low-sodium tamari

1 tbsp freshly squeezed lemon juice

3 cups cooked brown rice, to serve

½ cup chopped fresh cilantro leaves (optional), to garnish

For the spice blend

1 tbsp ground coriander

1 tbsp ground cumin

2 tsp paprika

1 tsp turmeric

1 tsp garam masala

½ tsp cayenne

Indian cuisine is simply magnificent, rich in exploding flavors and plant options. Chana masala means "spiced chickpeas" and is a popular spicy curry with a sour note. This simple version doesn't disappoint. Made from ingredients we always have on the shelf, it is a quick, go-to stew that can be whipped up at the end of the week, when supplies may be limited, to spice things up.

1   Prepare the spice blend. Place all spices in a small bowl and mix well. Set aside.

2   Heat a medium saucepan over medium-high heat. Once hot, sauté the onions with 1 to 2 tablespoons water—use just enough to avoid burning—until the onions are translucent. Add the hot pepper and cook an additional 3 to 5 minutes, until it softens. Add the garlic and ginger and sauté for 60 to 90 seconds, or until golden, taking care not to scorch.

3   Add the spice blend and stir to combine. Add the tomatoes and chickpeas and bring to a boil. Reduce the heat to low, stir to combine, and cover. Simmer for 15 minutes, stirring frequently. If the mixture becomes too thick while simmering, add up to ½ cup water, as needed, to avoid scorching.

4   Remove the pan from the heat. Add the tamari and lemon juice, and adjust to taste. Serve hot over rice and garnish with cilantro leaves, if desired.

✎ **NOTES:** To intensify the flavors, toast the cumin and coriander seeds and then crush them using a mortar and pestle or coffee grinder before adding to the spice blend.

Choose your peppers according to your tolerance for heat. Serrano chiles are considerably spicier than jalapeños.

This is a perfect recipe to batch-cook and freeze for later use when you need a hearty, last-minute meal.

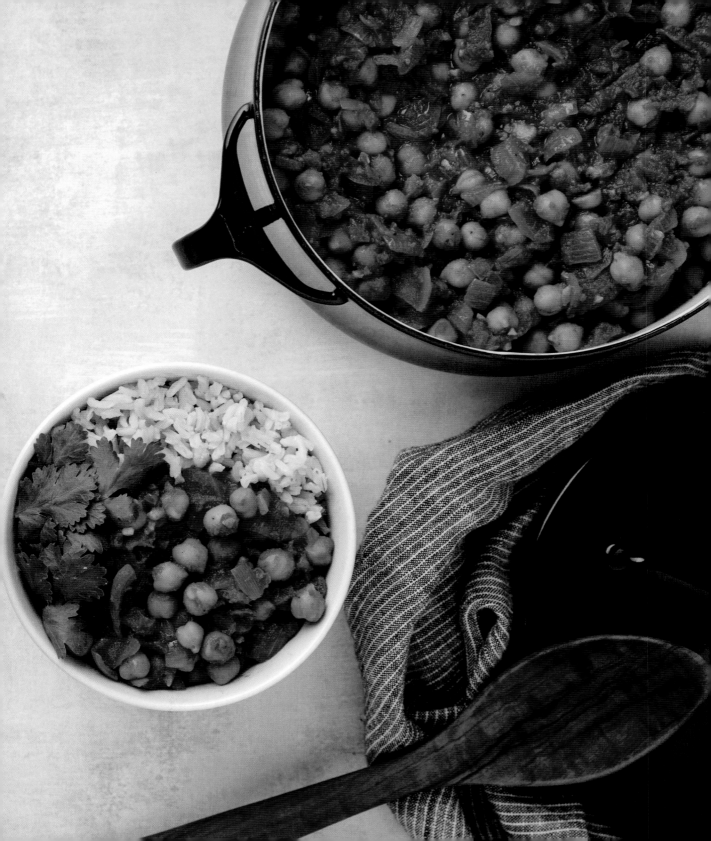

ROSEMARY POTATO-LEEK SOUP

PREP TIME: **15 MINUTES**
COOK TIME: **35 MINUTES**
YIELD: **8 CUPS**

INGREDIENTS

2 medium-large leeks

5–6 medium Yukon Gold potatoes, washed and chopped into 1-inch pieces

2 tbsp chopped fresh rosemary

4 cups **Simple Stock** (page 96) or low-sodium vegetable broth

1 cup unsweetened nondairy milk

2 tbsp nutritional yeast

2–3 tbsp low-sodium tamari, to taste

Freshly ground black pepper, to taste

Scallions, thinly sliced, to garnish

This is our take on the classic Welsh or French soup, but with a hint of rosemary to capture the essence of autumn. Delicate and comforting, creamy and smooth, this is a lovely soup to include in your regular repertoire.

1   To prepare the leeks, cut off the dark green tops and discard. Slice the leeks in half lengthwise. Cut off the root end, separate the leaves, and wash out any dirt under cold running water. Cut into ½-inch slices.

2   Heat a large stock pot over medium-high heat. Sauté the leeks with 3 to 4 tablespoons water or vegetable broth until softened and beginning to brown.

3   Use a little warm water to deglaze the pan and then add the potatoes, rosemary, and broth. Bring to a boil and then reduce heat, cover, and simmer for about 15 to 20 minutes, until potatoes are soft.

4   Remove from heat and add the nondairy milk, nutritional yeast, tamari, and black pepper. Purée with an immersion blender until creamy and smooth. (You may want to leave in some chunks of potatoes and leeks for texture or even remove a cup before blending to add back after the soup is puréed.)

5   Add the tamari and black pepper, as desired, and garnish with scallions. Serve hot.

MOROCCAN RED LENTIL SOUP
with Swiss Chard

PREP TIME: **20 MINUTES**
COOK TIME: **30 MINUTES**
YIELD: **8 CUPS**

INGREDIENTS

1 cup diced yellow onion

1 cup diced carrots

2 garlic cloves, minced

1 tsp ground cumin

1 tsp sweet paprika

½ tsp ground ginger

½ tsp ground turmeric

½ tsp red chili flakes

1 tbsp freshly squeezed lemon juice

1 (15oz) can diced tomatoes

1 cup dried red lentils, rinsed

6 cups **Simple Stock** (page 96) or
   low-sodium vegetable broth

1 bunch Swiss chard, stems
   removed, roughly chopped

1 tbsp low-sodium tamari

½ tsp liquid smoke

Lemon wedges, to serve

Freshly ground black pepper,
   to taste

Moroccan flavors infused with warm spices make for a delicious way to enjoy legumes and greens. Some notable nutrition perks of this recipe include the synergy of combining vitamin C–rich tomatoes and lemon juice with iron-rich lentils for optimal mineral absorption. Also, the black pepper boosts the bioavailability of the phytonutrient-rich turmeric.

1   Heat a large saucepan over medium-high heat. Dry sauté the onion and carrots with as little water as possible until the onions are translucent. (Use just enough water to avoid burning while allowing the vegetables to brown.) Add the garlic, cumin, paprika, ginger, turmeric, chili flakes, and lemon juice, and sauté for 30 to 60 seconds more.

2   Stir in the tomatoes, using the juice to scrape up the browned bits from the bottom of the pan. Cook for an additional minute. The liquid will reduce.

3   Add the lentils and broth. Bring to a boil, and then reduce the heat and simmer uncovered for 15 to 20 minutes, or until the lentils are desired tenderness.

4   Add the Swiss chard, tamari, and liquid smoke and cook for 3 to 5 minutes or until the chard begins to wilt. (Do not overcook.) Serve hot with a lemon wedge and black pepper to taste.

CREAM SOUP FORMULATOR

PREP TIME: **10 MINUTES**
COOK TIME: **15 MINUTES**
YIELD: **4–5 CUPS**

INGREDIENTS

For the soup

½ cup diced onion (optional)

2 cups low-sodium vegetable broth

2–3 cups chopped vegetables of choice

Fresh herbs of choice (optional)

For the cashew cream

¼ cup raw cashews (or hemp seeds)

2 tsp arrowroot powder or cornstarch

½ cup unsweetened nondairy milk

Dry herbs and spices of choice

This template for cream of vegetable soup involves three steps: cook the vegetables, purée or blend, and add a cashew cream to thicken. We use cashews for their mild flavor and creamy texture and arrowroot for its neutral flavor and ability to stand up to heat. You can substitute hemp seeds for nut allergies. There are countless combinations of vegetables, spices, and herbs, so experiment a little!

1   If using fresh onion or garlic, sauté the onion first until translucent and beginning to brown. Add the fresh garlic for the last 30 to 60 seconds. Avoid burning the garlic.

2   Add the vegetable broth and bring to a low simmer. Add your vegetables of choice and simmer, covered, for 5 minutes.

3   While the vegetables steam, make the cashew cream. In a blender or food processor, pulse the cashews with the arrowroot to a fine powder, but stop before it becomes a paste. Add the nondairy milk along with the spices and herbs of your choice, and blend well to mix.

4   After 5 minutes, remove ½ to ¾ cup vegetables (if you want to add whole pieces back to the creamed soup). Add the fresh herbs of your choice, if using, and use an immersion blender in the pan to purée the remaining vegetables.

5   Return to a simmer, stir in the cashew cream base, and continue heating for 3 to 5 minutes or until the desired consistency is achieved. Stir in any liquid flavor additions, such as lemon or lime juice, tamari, or mustard. Serve topped with reserved vegetables, if desired, and any additional garnishes.

✎ **NOTE:** Always pulse dry ingredients with cashews first to get a fine powder and then add the liquids. This avoids the need to soak the nuts to make them creamy.

CORN

1 garlic clove, minced

2 cups frozen corn kernels

½ tsp ground turmeric

½ tsp freshly ground black pepper

1 tbsp chopped flat-leaf (Italian) parsley

2 tsp low-sodium tamari

Squeeze of lime (optional), to serve

Sriracha or sliced jalapeño (optional), to serve

ASPARAGUS

1lb asparagus, trimmed and chopped

1 tsp Dijon mustard

2 tsp freshly squeezed lemon juice

1 tsp low-sodium tamari

1 tbsp basil chiffonade, to garnish

KABOCHA

2 cups cubed kabocha squash

1–2 tsp rubbed sage

1 tbsp low-sodium tamari

1 tsp molasses

1 tbsp black walnuts (optional), to garnish

BROCCOLI

2 cups broccoli florets

1 tbsp nutritional yeast

½ tsp garlic powder

½ tsp crushed red chili flakes

½ tsp freshly ground black pepper

1 tsp low-sodium tamari

1 tbsp Dijon mustard

2 tsp freshly squeezed lemon juice

ROASTED RED PEPPER

1 garlic clove, minced

3 roasted red bell peppers

½ tsp smoked paprika

¼ tsp ground chipotle powder

1 tsp nutritional yeast

1 tsp apple cider vinegar

1 tsp freshly squeezed lemon juice

2 tsp low-sodium tamari

TOMATO

1 (28oz) can fire-roasted tomatoes

½ tsp dried oregano

¼ tsp crushed red pepper flakes

2 tbsp minced fresh basil

2 tsp low-sodium tamari

1 tsp balsamic vinegar

1 tsp molasses

MUSHROOM

8oz gourmet mushroom mix, shiitake mushrooms, or baby bellas, sliced (sauté with onion)

1 tbsp minced fresh thyme

2 tsp freshly squeezed lemon juice

1 tbsp low-sodium tamari

CAULIFLOWER

2 cups chopped cauliflower florets

1½ tsp curry powder

1 tsp onion powder

¼ tsp garlic powder

¼ tsp freshly ground black pepper

1 tbsp low-sodium tamari

ZUCCHINI

2 garlic cloves, minced

2lb (about 4 cups) zucchini, chopped

1 tbsp pine nuts (pulse with cashews)

1 tbsp minced fresh basil, plus more to garnish

1 tbsp low-sodium tamari

½ tsp freshly ground black pepper

MAMA'S BUTTER BEAN SOUP

PREP TIME: **20 MINUTES**
COOK TIME: **40 MINUTES**
YIELD: **3 QUARTS**

INGREDIENTS

2 cups diced yellow onion

3 cups diced carrots

2½ cups sliced celery

4 sprigs fresh thyme

3–5 garlic cloves, quartered

¾ cup white wine

1 (15oz) can diced tomatoes

2 (15oz) cans low-sodium butter beans, drained and rinsed

1 (15oz) can low-sodium cannellini beans, drained and rinsed

1 cup chopped cabbage (green or red)

4 cups chopped kale

¼ cup chopped parsley, to garnish

2 tbsp sliced scallions, to garnish

1–2 tbsp freshly squeezed lemon juice, to serve

Ray's mom, Lois, is an amazing cook. Her fridge and pantry are always stocked with goodies for decadent, healthy meals. Her soup has been a hit with many of our clients, and we both love it, too. Cruciferous vegetables, creamy butter beans, crisp white wine, and heavenly herbs come together in a perfect blend. It's easy to make, easy to store, and absolutely wonderful to eat.

1 Heat a large saucepan or Dutch oven over medium-high heat. Once hot, sauté the onions, carrots, celery, and thyme with 1 to 2 tablespoons water for 2 to 3 minutes or until beginning to brown. Add the garlic and sauté for 1 to 2 minutes more, taking care not to scorch.

2 Add the wine, reduce the heat to medium-low, cover, and simmer for 10 to 15 minutes.

3 Remove the thyme stems. (Most of the leaves should have fallen off, but strip any that remain and add them back in.) Add the tomatoes, butter beans, cannellini beans, and 8 cups water. Cover and return to a boil. Remove the lid and simmer 10 minutes more. Add the cabbage and simmer 5 minutes more.

4 Add the kale and simmer until it is just wilted. Serve hot with parsley, scallions, and lemon juice.

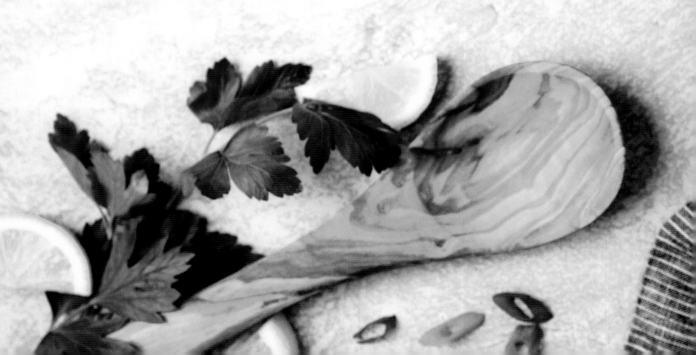

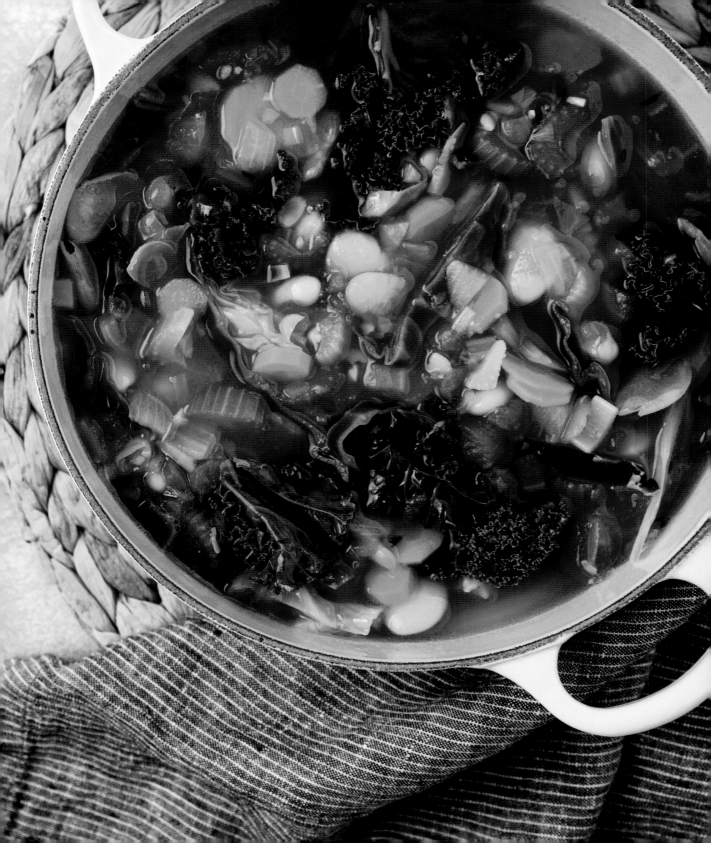

BRUNSWICK STEW

PREP TIME: **10 MINUTES**
COOK TIME: **45 MINUTES**
YIELD: **8 CUPS**

INGREDIENTS

1 (20oz) can young green jackfruit, drained and rinsed (net 10oz drained)

2 tbsp barbecue sauce (preferably a North Carolina-style, vinegar-based variety; see note.)

1 tsp liquid smoke

2 cups chopped sweet yellow onion

1 tsp extra virgin olive oil

3 garlic cloves, minced

1 (6oz) can tomato paste

1 tsp smoked paprika

2 tbsp low-sodium tamari

2 tbsp anchovy-free Worcestershire sauce

1 (14oz) can fire-roasted diced tomatoes

1 (16oz) bag frozen, fire-roasted yellow corn (or frozen yellow corn, skillet roasted)

1 (16oz) bag frozen butter beans

2 cups **Simple Stock** (page 96) or low-sodium vegetable broth

1 tsp molasses

Freshly ground black pepper, to taste

Despite the fun debate on where Brunswick stew originated (possibly Brunswick County, Virginia; Brunswick, Georgia; or Braunschweig, Germany), it is commonly enjoyed in the South. Traditionally, this is a thick, tomato-based stew with local beans, vegetables, and small game meat; we swap in young green jackfruit to healthfully mimic a meaty texture in this hearty, flavorful, and satisfying stew.

1 To prepare the jackfruit, drain the liquid from the can and rinse. The pie-shaped slices have a dense core near the pointy end and are more fibrous at the wider end. Using the palm of your hand or a flat bench scraper, smash the jackfruit slices. There might be a few tiny seeds, which can be removed. The outer portion should look like shredded pork or chicken, but the inner portion may need a little more smashing to pull apart. Once it is all shredded and flat, use paper towels or a cloth to remove as much water as possible (see note).

2 In a medium bowl, combine the jackfruit, barbecue sauce, and liquid smoke. Set aside to marinate for 30 to 40 minutes.

3 In a large saucepan, sauté the onions with a splash of water over medium heat for 2 to 3 minutes or until tender. Move the onions to the side of the pan and add the olive oil in the center. Add the garlic to the oil and sauté until golden, taking care not to let it burn. Add the jackfruit and marinade to the pan along with the tomato paste, smoked paprika, tamari, and Worcestershire sauce. Sauté for 3 to 4 minutes.

4 Add the tomatoes, roasted corn, butter beans, vegetable broth, and molasses. Simmer over medium heat, uncovered, for about 30 minutes. Sprinkle with black pepper, if using, and serve hot.

✎ **NOTES:** If you have a vacuum sealer, place a folded paper towel with jackfruit in the bag after the water has been removed manually, as described in step 1. Then use the vacuum sealer to remove even more of the brine. Remove the wet paper towels, add the barbecue sauce and liquid smoke, and use the vacuum sealer again to push flavors in deeper.

If you cannot find a North Carolina–style, vinegar-based barbecue sauce, add a tablespoon of apple cider vinegar before serving for more acidity.

ROASTED ROOT BISQUE

PREP TIME: **20 MINUTES**
COOK TIME: **25 MINUTES**
YIELD: **6 CUPS**

INGREDIENTS

2 cups diced parsnips

2 cups diced carrots

2 cups diced yellow onion

2 cups peeled and diced sweet
potato (see note)

1 tsp olive oil (optional)

¼ cup raw cashews

¼ cup unsweetened nondairy milk

2 tsp minced fresh thyme

2 tsp minced fresh rosemary

2 garlic cloves, sliced thin

6 cups **Simple Stock** (page 96) or
low-sodium vegetable broth

Salt and freshly ground black
pepper, to taste

1 tbsp roasted pepitas (optional),
to garnish

Root vegetables grow underground, where they absorb myriad minerals, including manganese, copper, and potassium. Roasting these hearty vegetables brings out their sweetness via the caramelization process. Blended together with plant milk and seasonings, this soup is soothing, creamy, and a cozy representative of autumn.

1 Preheat the oven to 450°F. Line a baking sheet with parchment paper or a silicone baking mat. In a medium bowl, toss the parsnips, carrots, onions, and sweet potato with olive oil, if using. (A little olive oil goes a long way, so it's completely optional.) Spread the vegetables on the prepared baking sheet and roast for 20 minutes, taking care not to burn the smaller vegetables, particularly the onions.

2 Meanwhile, place the cashews in a blender. Pulse until a fine powder forms, but not long enough to create a paste. Scrape the corners of the blender with a spatula to make sure all the powder is free. Add the nondairy milk and blend until fully combined and creamy. Set aside.

3 In a stock pot over medium-high heat, sauté the thyme, rosemary, and garlic with a splash of water for 30 to 60 seconds. Add half of the roasted vegetables and continue to sauté for 2 minutes more, adding vegetable broth as needed to keep the pan moist.

4 Add the remaining vegetable broth, cover, and simmer for 5 minutes. Purée well with an immersion blender, or carefully transfer in batches to a blender and blend until smooth. Taste and season with salt and pepper.

5 Add most of the reserved roasted vegetables to the bisque, saving some to garnish the bowl, if desired. Top each bowl with the roasted vegetable garnish, a drizzle of the cashew cream, and the roasted pepitas, if desired.

✎ **NOTES:** If sweet potato is too sweet, butternut squash can be used instead.

The smoother the better, and while not necessary, a chinois strainer can be used to make the bisque incredibly smooth.

SPICY THAI VEGETABLE CHOWDER

PREP TIME: **15 MINUTES**
COOK TIME: **30 MINUTES**
YIELD: **6 CUPS**

INGREDIENTS

½ tsp coriander seeds

1 medium yellow onion, diced

2 garlic cloves, minced

1 tbsp minced fresh ginger

2 tbsp finely chopped lemongrass

1–4 Thai chiles, deseeded and minced, to taste

1 cup diced carrots

1 cup diced red bell pepper

½ cup **Simple Stock** (page 96) or low-sodium vegetable broth

½ tsp crushed red pepper flakes (optional)

4 cups frozen corn kernels, thawed, divided

2 cups plain coconut water

1 cup unsweetened nondairy milk

2 cups sliced oyster mushrooms

1 tsp low-sodium tamari

¼ cup minced fresh cilantro leaves

¼ cup freshly squeezed lime juice

A chowder is defined as a thick soup or stew, commonly made with seafood, vegetables, potatoes, onions, and seasonings. Here, oyster mushrooms and sweet corn take center stage and are infused with classic Thai flavors of lemongrass, ginger, and lime in a creamy, spicy chowder that is brimming with texture and complexity.

1   In a large pot, lightly toast the coriander seeds over medium heat for 30 to 60 seconds. Add the onions, garlic, ginger, lemongrass, and chiles, and sauté over medium heat, stirring often, for 3 to 5 minutes. (Add a small amount of water or broth if the pan gets too dry.) Add the carrots, bell pepper, and vegetable broth and cook, stirring often, for 3 to 5 minutes more.

2   Add the red pepper flakes, if using, 2 cups corn kernels, coconut water, and nondairy milk. Bring to a boil over high heat. Cover, reduce the heat to low, and simmer for 10 minutes.

3   While the soup simmers, sauté the oyster mushrooms with tamari in a separate medium pan until the mushrooms release their liquid, 3 to 5 minutes.

4   Using an immersion blender, carefully blend the chowder until smooth and creamy. Stir in the remaining 2 cups corn kernels and sautéed oyster mushrooms, and simmer over medium-low heat for 5 minutes more.

5   Stir in the cilantro and lime juice. Remove from heat and serve hot.

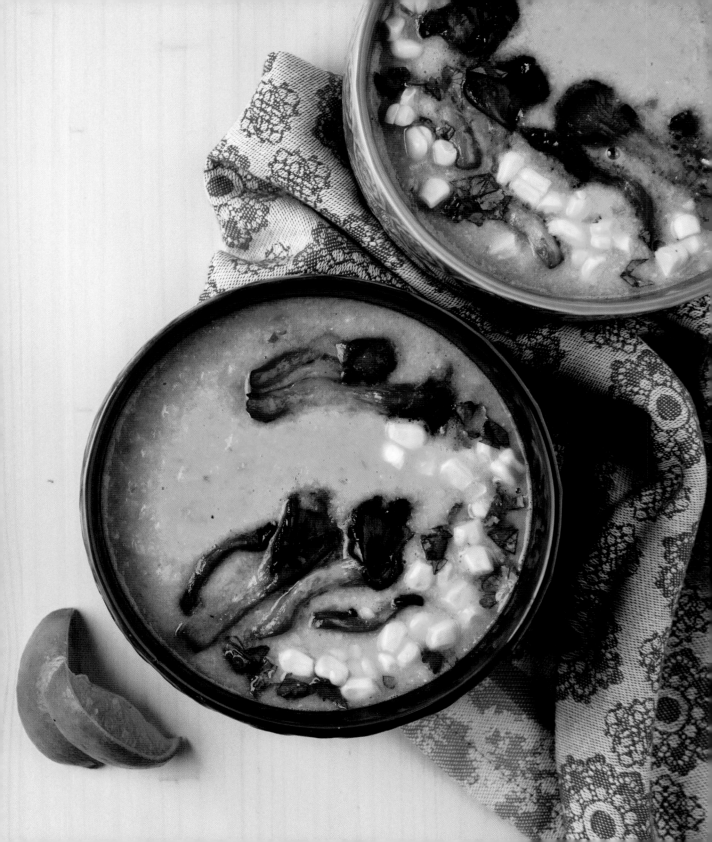

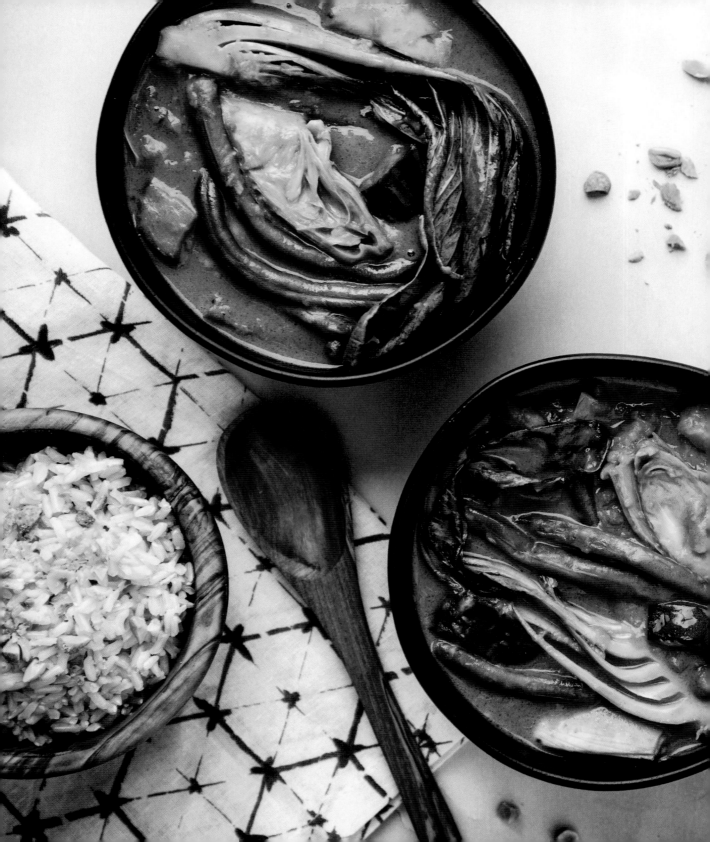

KARE-KARENG GULAY
(Filipino Peanut Vegetable Stew)

PREP TIME: **20 MINUTES**
COOK TIME: **30 MINUTES**
YIELD: **8 CUPS**

INGREDIENTS

1 tbsp annatto (achiote) powder

1 cup chopped sweet yellow onion (about 1 onion)

3 garlic cloves, minced

1 medium Chinese or Japanese eggplant, cut in rounds or quartered if larger diameter

1 cup long beans, cut into 3-in lengths (or green beans)

1 cup cubed winter squash (butternut, acorn, or kabocha)

4 cups **Simple Stock** (page 96) or low-sodium vegetable broth, divided

½ cup smooth unsweetened peanut butter

4–5 baby baby bok choy, quartered

1 cup canned quartered artichoke hearts, in water, rinsed

1 tbsp molasses

3 tbsp low-sodium tamari

½ tsp liquid smoke

Cooked rice (optional), to serve

½ cup chopped fresh-roasted peanuts, to garnish

This traditional Filipino stew tastes similar to peanut satay and is colored with annatto, a deep rusty orange, carotenoid-rich food coloring derived from the seeds of the achiote tree. The decadent array of textures and flavors from this unique combination of vegetables, swimming in peanutty goodness, translates to an unforgettable stew. Serve over rice for a super-satisfying meal.

1 In a small bowl, mix the annatto powder with 3 tablespoons water and set aside.

2 Heat a large saucepan or Dutch oven over medium-high heat. Once hot, sauté the onions with as little water as possible, just enough to avoid burning, until the onions are translucent. Add the garlic and sauté for 30 to 60 seconds, or until golden, being careful not to scorch.

3 Stir in the eggplant, long beans, squash, and 1 cup broth. Bring to a boil, and then reduce the heat to medium-low. Partially cover and cook for 7 to 10 minutes, stirring occasionally, until the squash begins to soften and the eggplant is translucent.

4 Add the annatto mixture, peanut butter, and remaining 3 cups broth. Increase the heat to bring to a boil, and then reduce the heat to medium-low and simmer for 10 to 15 minutes. Add the baby bok choy and artichoke hearts. Cover and cook for another 4 to 5 minutes until bok choy has softened. Stir in the molasses, tamari, and liquid smoke.

5 Serve hot over rice, if using, and top with chopped peanuts as a garnish.

✎ **NOTE:** Artichoke hearts are used in place of the harder-to-find banana flowers traditionally used in this dish. Feel free to try them if you are able to find these beautiful, exotic plants.

BLACK BEAN AND KALE CHILI

PREP TIME: **10 MINUTES**
COOK TIME: **50 MINUTES**
YIELD: **10 CUPS**

INGREDIENTS

1½ cups diced yellow onion, divided

3 garlic cloves, minced

2 (15oz) cans low-sodium black beans, drained

1 (15oz) can red kidney beans, drained

1 (28oz) can fire-roasted diced tomatoes

2 tbsp chili powder

2 tsp ground cumin

¼ tsp cayenne

2½ cups **Simple Stock** (page 96) or low-sodium vegetable broth

1 (6oz) can tomato paste

2–3 cups chopped kale

Everyone needs a go-to chili recipe that can be made without forethought and with ingredients that reside in your kitchen as staples. This recipe is the perfect candidate. It's also a great option for taking to a family and friends gathering. Who doesn't like a hearty bowl of chili that will stick to your ribs? Spicy hot, hearty, and chunky, this chili is one of our favorite ways to tuck away those daily beans and greens.

1   Heat a large saucepan or Dutch oven over medium-high heat. Once hot, sauté 1 cup onion with 1 to 2 tablespoons water—just enough to avoid burning—until the onions are translucent. Add the garlic and sauté for 60 to 90 seconds or until golden, taking care not to scorch.

2   Add the black beans, kidney beans, diced tomatoes, chili powder, cumin, cayenne, broth, and tomato paste. Stir to combine. Bring to a boil. Once boiling, lower heat, cover, and simmer for 40 to 50 minutes.

3   Add the kale during last 15 minutes of cooking. Serve hot, garnished with the remaining ½ cup onion. It also makes a great topping over black rice, quinoa, a baked potato, or a bed of greens.

SATISFYING SMOKY LENTIL STEW

PREP TIME: **10 MINUTES**
COOK TIME: **50 MINUTES**
YIELD: **6 CUPS**

INGREDIENTS

1½ cups chopped yellow onion

1½ cups chopped red bell pepper

2 garlic cloves, minced

4 cups **Simple Stock** (page 96), low-sodium vegetable broth or water, divided

1½ tbsp chili powder

1 tsp ground cumin

1 tsp smoked paprika

½ tsp ground chipotle powder

¼ tsp crushed red chili flakes

2 cups dried red lentils, rinsed

1 (28oz) can fire-roasted crushed tomatoes (plain is fine, too)

1 (15oz) can chickpeas, drained and rinsed

2 tbsp freshly squeezed lemon (or lime) juice

1 tsp lemon (or lime) zest

¼ cup chopped fresh cilantro (or Italian parsley), to garnish

Salt and freshly ground black pepper, to taste

This is a perfect one-pot dish to feed a family or batch-cook ahead of time to last all week. With smoky seasonings and plenty of nutritious legumes, this stew is satiating and simple. Serve on its own or over a baked potato or bowl of whole grains.

1 In a large pot, sauté the onions, bell pepper, and garlic in ½ cup vegetable broth over medium-high heat until the onions are translucent, about 5 minutes. Let them brown, but add more broth, as needed, to avoid burning. Add the chili powder, cumin, paprika, chipotle powder, and red chili flakes, and cook for an additional minute.

2 Add the lentils, crushed tomatoes, remaining 3½ cups vegetable broth, and chickpeas. Partially cover and bring to a boil. Once boiling, reduce the heat and simmer, stirring occasionally, until lentils are soft, about 30 minutes.

3 Stir in the lemon juice and zest, and sprinkle with cilantro leaves. Taste and season with salt and pepper. Serve hot.

GUAY TIEW TOM YUM

PREP TIME: **20 MINUTES**
COOK TIME: **30 MINUTES**
YIELD: **6 CUPS**

INGREDIENTS

1 shallot, sliced

½ cup sliced shiitake mushrooms

4 cups coconut water

3 garlic cloves, sliced

4 kaffir lime leaves

2-in piece lemongrass, smashed and sliced diagonally in pieces large enough to pick out

2-in piece galangal (Thai ginger), sliced

2–4 Thai chiles, slit on one side to release flavor

2 tbsp chili paste

1 bunch shimeji (beech) mushrooms, base trimmed

½ cup sliced baby bella mushrooms (or oyster, enoki, white button, or other mushrooms)

½ cup halved cherry tomatoes

4 tbsp freshly squeezed lime juice

1 tsp molasses

½ tsp **Magic Mushroom Powder** (page 242)

2 cups raw zucchini noodles or cooked rice noodles

½ cup cilantro leaves, to garnish

Lime slices, to garnish

A much-beloved, hot-and-sour soup in Thailand, this is one of our favorite ways to combine these authentic flavors. Spicy Thai chilis; sour kaffir limes, lemongrass, and lime juice; sweet molasses; and, of course, a strapping dose of umami from the mushrooms in our Magic Mushroom Powder make this soup scrumptious. We also added noodles—despite fraying from tradition—because, well, who doesn't like another excuse to slurp up noodles?

1   Heat a large saucepan or Dutch oven over medium-high heat. Once hot, sauté the shallot and mushrooms with as little water as possible—just enough to avoid burning—for about 3 minutes.

2   Add the coconut water, garlic, kaffir lime leaves, lemongrass, galangal, and Thai chiles and bring to a simmer for 5 minutes. Add the chili paste and stir to mix.

3   Add the shimeji mushrooms, baby bella mushrooms, tomatoes, and lime juice. Let it simmer for 10 minutes and taste to adjust the sweet-sour balance. Start by adding 1 teaspoon molasses. This should be close, but a little more may be necessary.

4   Add the raw zucchini noodles or cooked rice noodles and simmer for 2 to 4 minutes to heat. Before eating, remove the lemongrass, galangal slices, and lime leaves. Garnish with cilantro and sliced lime. Serve hot.

NOTE: For a creamy version, reduce the coconut water to 3 cups and replace with cashew cream. To make the cashew cream, pulse ¼ cup raw cashews in a blender until a powder forms. Add ¾ cup coconut water and ½ tsp arrowroot powder. Blend until well-combined. Add to the soup at the end of step 4 and simmer for 2 to 3 minutes until slightly thickened.

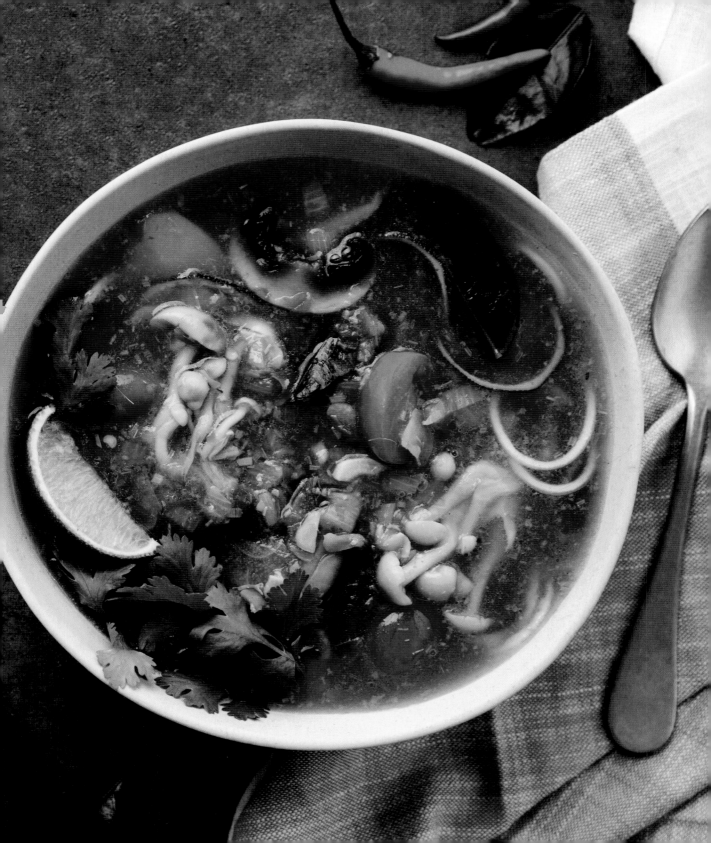

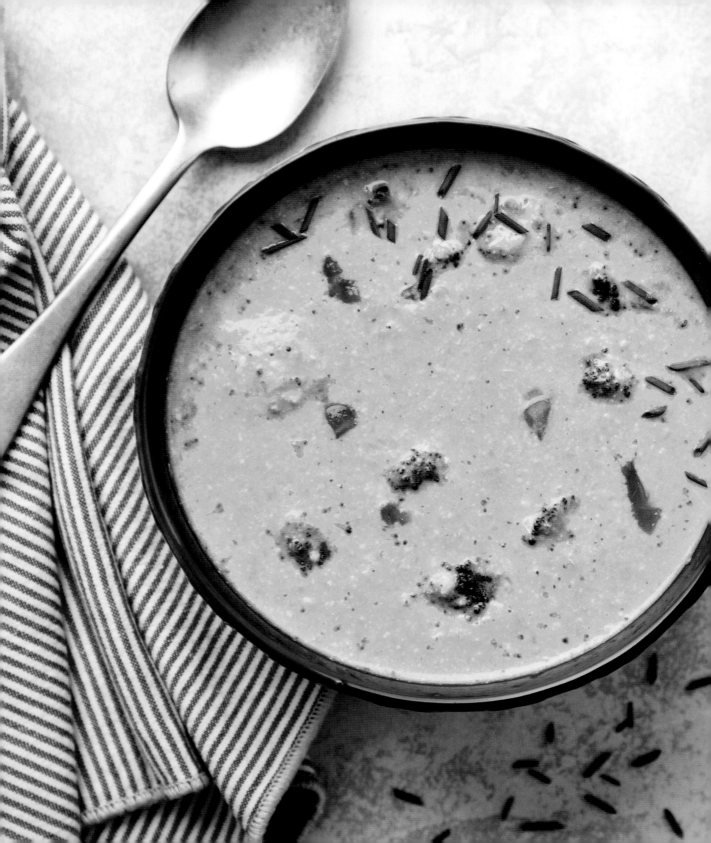

RO-TEL BROCCOLI BISQUE

PREP TIME: **10 MINUTES**
COOK TIME: **20 MINUTES**
YIELD: **6 CUPS**

INGREDIENTS

2 cups **Simple Stock** (page 96) or low-sodium vegetable broth

2 cups bite-size broccoli florets

1½ cups **Chipotle Butternut Cheesy Sauce** (page 239)

1 (10oz) can Original RO-TEL Diced Tomatoes and Green Chilies (or choose hot or mild, if preferred)

2 tsp arrowroot powder

Chives, chopped, to garnish

RO-TEL dip began as a 1949 Texas marketing campaign to promote a canned diced tomato and chili product by Carl Roettelle. By the 70s, it was a mainstay party food all across the South. All one needed was a block of Velveeta (technically not cheese), a can of RO-TEL Tomatoes and Chilies, and a heat source. (We used the microwave.) This dairy-free soup re-creates the flavors of that addictive dip using delicious whole foods. We called it "bisque" just to sound fancy, but we think you and the kids are going to love it. Grab a spoon.

1 In a medium saucepan, bring the vegetable broth to a boil. Reduce the heat to medium-low, add the broccoli florets, and cover. Allow to steam for 5 minutes.

2 Remove 1½ cups broccoli florets and set aside, leaving about ½ cup broccoli behind in the pan. Using an immersion blender, blend the remaining broccoli and stock. (It doesn't need to be fully blended, as it just adds flavor and smaller bits of broccoli to the soup.)

3 Add the Chipotle Butternut Cheesy Sauce and RO-TEL to the pan. Stir for an even consistency. Heat over medium heat until simmering, but not to a full boil.

4 In a small bowl or measuring cup, mix the arrowroot powder with 1 tablespoon cold water to form a slurry. Slowly pour the slurry into the simmering soup, stirring constantly. Stir for 2 to 3 minutes until it thickens.

5 Fold in the reserved 1½ cups broccoli florets. Cook for 1 to 2 minutes until fully heated, but don't boil. Garnish with chives and serve immediately.

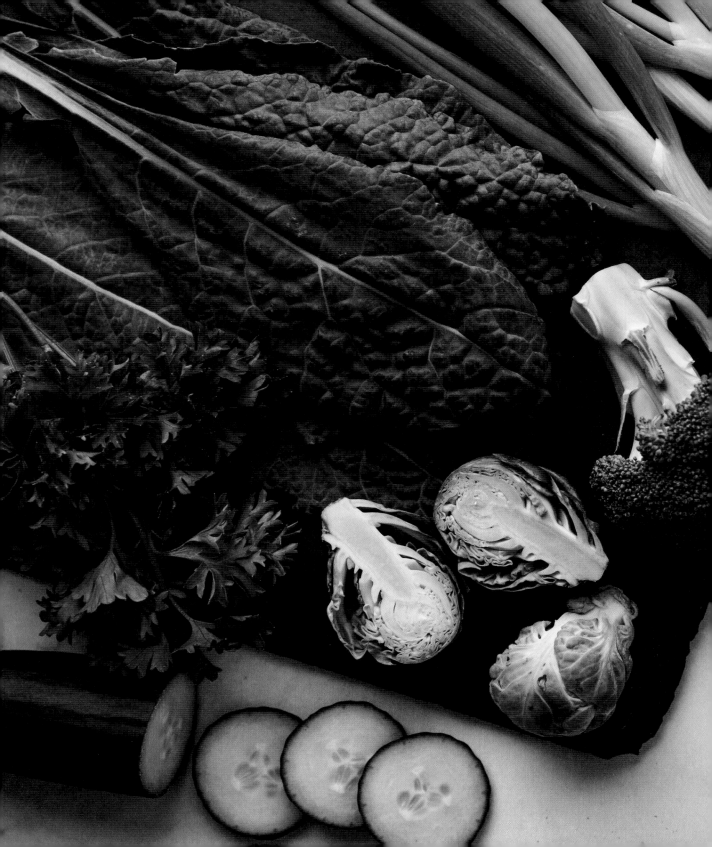

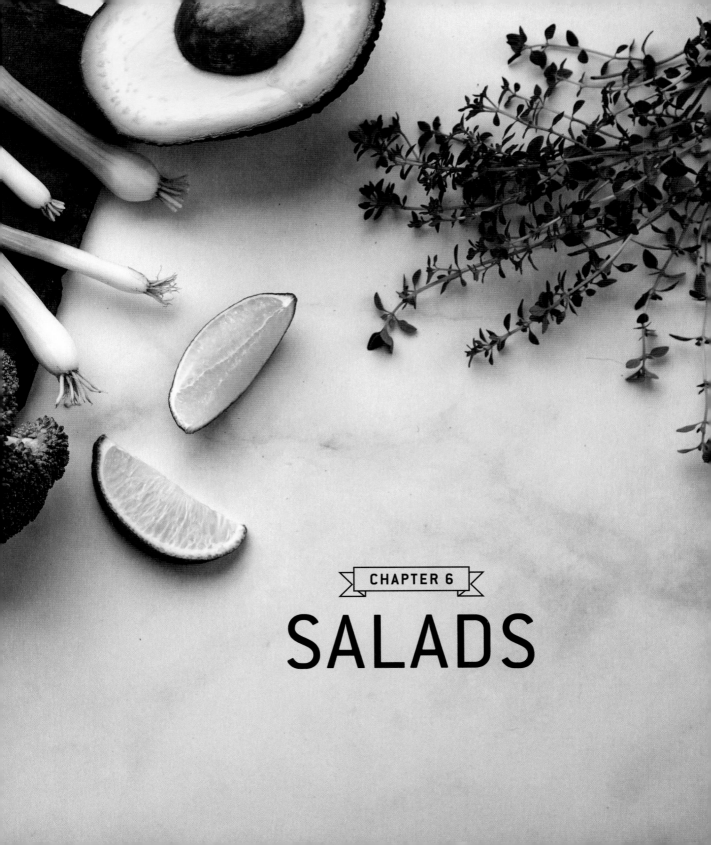

CHAPTER 6

SALADS

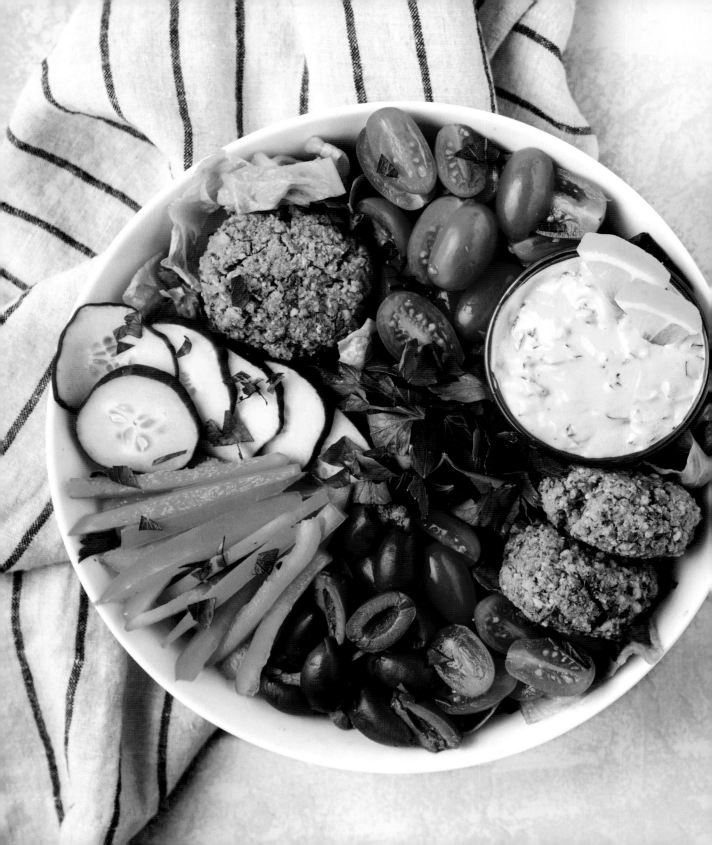

FALAFEL SALAD
with Lemon-Garlic Tahini Dressing

PREP TIME: **15 MINUTES**
COOK TIME: **NONE**
YIELD: **2 SERVINGS**

This bowl of veggies is the perfect bed of freshness for our warm, toasty Baked Falafel recipe. Light, healthy, and super satisfying, it's a delcious way to enjoy traditional Middle Eastern flavors.

INGREDIENTS

1 head romaine lettuce, chopped

1 cup halved grape or cherry tomatoes

1 cup sliced cucumber

1 cup sliced red bell pepper

¼ cup pitted Kalamata olives

4–8 **Baked Falafel** (page 176)

For the dressing

4 tbsp tahini

2 tbsp freshly squeezed lemon juice

1 tsp minced garlic

¼ tsp smoked paprika

1 tsp minced flat-leaf (Italian) parsley

1 In a small bowl, combine all dressing ingredients, except the parsley. Stir until well combined, adding 4 to 6 tablespoons warm water as needed to achieve the desired thickness. Add the parsley and stir to combine.

2 To assemble the salads, divide the lettuce, tomatoes, cucumber, bell pepper, and olives evenly between two salad bowls. Add 2 to 4 falafel to each salad, drizzle with the dressing, and serve.

GREEN APPLE AND BRUSSELS SPROUT SLAW

PREP TIME: **10 MINUTES**
COOK TIME: **NONE**
YIELD: **2–4 SERVINGS**

INGREDIENTS

1½ cups shredded Brussels sprouts

½ cup chopped red cabbage

1 large green apple, cut into matchsticks

¼ cup dried tart cherries, cranberries, or raisins (no added sugar)

1 tbsp chopped raw pecans, to garnish

Freshly ground black pepper, to taste

For the dressing

¼ cup raw pecans

1 tbsp nutritional yeast

2 tsp freshly squeezed lemon juice

2 tsp maple syrup

½ tsp low-sodium tamari

½ tsp Dijon mustard

Brussels sprouts, one of the most hated vegetables as a child, often become one of the most beloved as an adult. Their cruciferous classification makes them a top-Triangle food. In fact, Brussels sprouts provide a high dose of cancer-protective glucosinolates, help reduce cholesterol levels, and are an excellent source of fiber and vitamins C and K. Combined with crisp green apple, crunchy cabbage, and tart cherries and drizzled with a balanced sweet-and-sour pecan dressing, this is a simple and sassy way to include more of these health-promoting veggies.

1   Arrange the shredded Brussels sprouts, cabbage, apple, and dried cherries in a serving bowl.

2   To make the dressing, in a blender, pulse ¼ cup pecans with the nutritional yeast until it becomes a fine powder. Add the lemon juice, maple syrup, tamari, and mustard, and blend until smooth and well combined.

3   Pour the dressing over the salad and toss to combine. Top with 1 tablespoon chopped pecans and black pepper, to taste. Serve immediately.

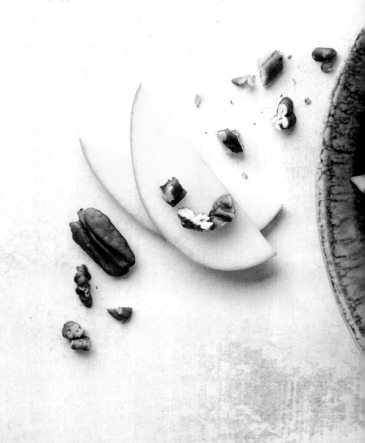

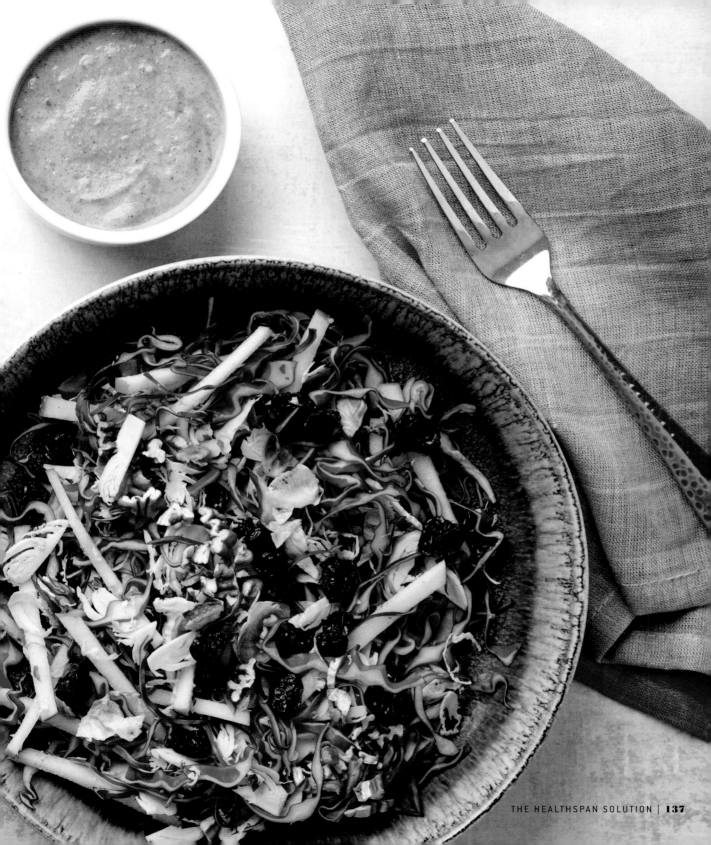

FRESH MARKET SALAD
with Creamy Ranch Dressing

PREP TIME: **20 MINUTES**
COOK TIME: **5 MINUTES**
YIELD: **2 SERVINGS**

INGREDIENTS

4 cups spring mix

2 cups shredded Brussels sprouts

¼ cup chopped sun-dried tomatoes (not packed in oil)

1 cup sliced fresh tomatoes

1 cup broccoli florets

1 cup sliced cucumber

1 cup shredded carrots

1 cup shredded beets

1 cup jicama matchsticks

1 tbsp raw sunflower seeds

For the dressing

½ cup raw cashews

½ cup unsweetened nondairy milk

1¾ tsp apple cider vinegar

1 tsp freshly squeezed lemon juice

1 tsp finely chopped fresh flat-leaf (Italian) parsley or ¼ tsp dried parsley

½ tsp low-sodium tamari

¼ tsp dried dill

¼ tsp freshly ground black pepper

⅛ tsp onion powder

⅛ tsp garlic powder

For the mushroom topping (optional)

1 cup sliced shiitake mushrooms

1 tsp low-sodium tamari

⅛ tsp garlic powder

This salad was inspired by one of our favorite dishes at The Wild Cow, our favorite restaurant in Nashville. We schedule all our flights around its store hours so we can stop by on the way to and from the airport. All the nutrition, color, flavor, and texture elements are represented in this one bowl.

1   Divide the spring mix and Brussels sprouts evenly between two large salad bowls, and arrange the remaining salad ingredients on top.

2   To make the dressing, in a blender, pulse the cashews into a fine powder. Add the remaining dressing ingredients and blend until smooth and well combined.

3   If making the optional mushroom topping, heat a large saucepan over medium-high heat. Once hot, add the mushrooms and cook until their liquid is released, 3 to 5 minutes. In a small bowl, stir together the tamari, garlic powder, and 1 tablespoon water. Pour the mixture over the mushrooms, stir to combine, and wait for mushrooms to absorb the liquid. Remove from the heat and add to the salad.

4   Pour the dressing over the salads and enjoy immediately.

✎ **NOTE:** This makes two huge and hearty salads, so you can halve everything if you are making it for one. It also makes extra dressing that can be stored in the refrigerator for use over the week.

GREEK QUINOA SALAD
with Olive and Balsamic Dressing

PREP TIME: **15 MINUTES**
COOK TIME: **NONE**
YIELD: **2 SERVINGS**

INGREDIENTS

2 cups cooked quinoa, fully cooled

2 cups chopped romaine lettuce

1 cup chopped English (hothouse) cucumber

1 cup chopped red bell pepper

¼ cup chopped red onion

¼ cup sliced radishes

½ avocado, chopped

Freshly ground black pepper, to serve

Lemon wedges, to serve

For the dressing

4–5 Kalamata olives, pitted

1 tsp Dijon mustard

1 tsp freshly squeezed lemon juice

2 tsp balsamic vinegar

¼ tsp garlic powder

¼ cup + 2 tbsp unsweetened nondairy milk

Blending olives into a dressing lends a robust, bright, briny flavor explosion, which makes for a fresh, light Greek salad when tossed with crisp lettuce, radishes, bell peppers, and cucumbers. Add some creamy avocado and fluffy quinoa and you have a substantial, satisfying meal.

1 Divide the quinoa evenly between two large salad bowls. On top of the quinoa, arrange the lettuce, cucumber, bell pepper, onions, radish, and avocado.

2 In a blender, combine all the dressing ingredients and blend until smooth, about 30 seconds.

3 Drizzle the dressing over each salad, toss to combine, and serve immediately with black pepper and a lemon wedge.

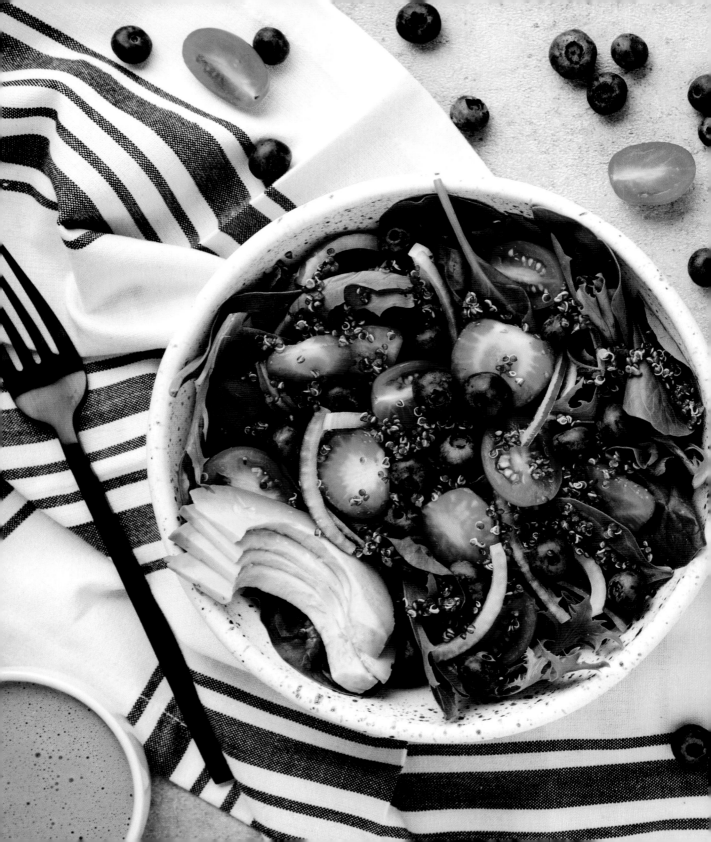

QUINOA BERRY SALAD
with Creamy Balsamic Dressing

PREP TIME: **15 MINUTES**
COOK TIME: **NONE**
YIELD: **2 SERVINGS**

INGREDIENTS

4 cups mixed salad greens or arugula

1 cup cooked red quinoa, fully cooled

½ cup sliced strawberries

½ cup blueberries

½ cup halved grape or cherry tomatoes

¼ cup thinly sliced red onion

½ avocado, sliced

For the dressing

½ cup raw cashews

½ cup unsweetened nondairy milk

½ cup balsamic vinegar

2 tbsp diced shallot

2 tsp Dijon mustard

This is one more way to enjoy every color of the rainbow in a single delectable dish. While any colored quinoa is nutritionally exceptional, the red variety contains an extra dose of anti-inflammatory and antioxidant phytonutrients known as *betacyanins*, the compound responsible for the deep red coloring. This toothsome salad is filled with fresh ingredients and topped with a sweet balsamic-Dijon dressing.

1   To make the dressing, in a blender, pulse the cashews until ground to a fine powder but not a paste, approximately 30 seconds. Add the remaining dressing ingredients and blend until smooth.

2   Divide the greens and quinoa evenly between two large salad bowls. Top each bowl with the strawberries, blueberries, tomatoes, red onions, and avocado slices. Drizzle with dressing and serve immediately.

CHOPPED ASIAN SALAD
with Spicy Peanut Dressing

PREP TIME: **25 MINUTES**
COOK TIME: **5 MINUTES**
YIELD: **2 SERVINGS**

INGREDIENTS

For the mushrooms

½ cup sliced shiitake mushrooms

1 tsp low-sodium tamari

¼ tsp garlic powder

For the dressing

¼ cup fresh roasted peanuts

2 tbsp unsweetened nondairy milk

1 tbsp freshly squeezed lime juice

1½ tsp Sriracha

1½ tsp low-sodium tamari

1 tsp seasoned rice vinegar

¼ tsp grated fresh ginger

½ tsp toasted sesame oil

For the salad

1 cup cooked black forbidden rice

1 cup chopped mango

¼ cup sliced scallions

½ cup shredded carrot

½ cup chopped red pepper

½ cup shredded daikon

½ cup cooked edamame

1 cup chopped romaine lettuce

½ cup chopped purple cabbage

½ cup chopped napa cabbage

1 tbsp chopped peanuts, to garnish

Black forbidden rice offers an enigmatic name and history, a distinctive texture, and a rich phytonutrient profile. Forbidden to the people because it was reserved for an ancient emperor in China and prized for its anthocyanin content more recently, this grain is special. Together with other Asian-inspired ingredients, this salad is fresh and flavorful, with plenty of texture and a decadent peanut butter dressing.

1 Prepare the mushroom topping. In a medium saucepan over medium-high heat, sauté the shiitake mushrooms with 1 to 2 tablespoons water until tender. In a small bowl, stir together the tamari, garlic powder, and 1 tablespoon water. Once the mushrooms begin to release water and reduce in size, add the tamari mixture to the pan. Let some of the water evaporate and absorb into the mushrooms. Remove from the heat and set aside.

2 Prepare the dressing. In a blender, pulse the peanuts into a fine powder. Add the remaining dressing ingredients and 2 tablespoons warm water and blend until smooth. For a thinner consistency, add more warm water or nondairy milk.

3 Assemble the salad. Place all the salad ingredients in a wide, shallow bowl along with the cooked shiitakes. Pour the dressing over top and sprinkle with chopped peanuts, if desired. Toss to combine and serve immediately.

✎ **NOTE:** Prepare black forbidden rice on the stove, in a rice cooker, or in a pressure cooker. You can use another long-grain rice, if preferred.

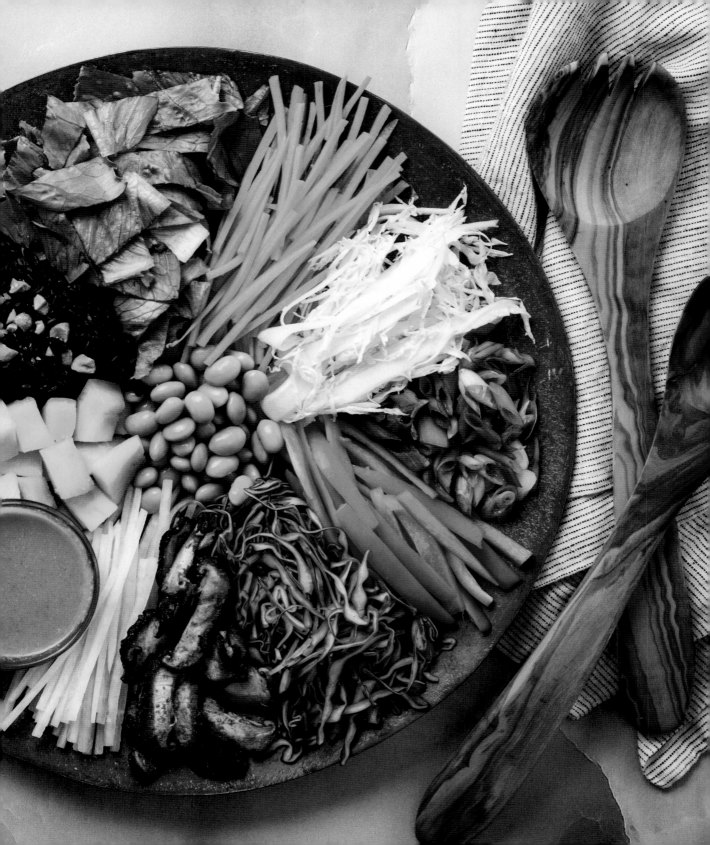

LEMON-TAHINI BROCCOLI SLAW

PREP TIME: **10 MINUTES**
COOK TIME: **NONE**
YIELD: **6 CUPS**

INGREDIENTS

4 tbsp tahini

2 tbsp + 1½ tsp freshly squeezed lemon juice

2 garlic cloves, minced

2 tsp low-sodium tamari

¼ tsp freshly ground black pepper

12oz broccoli slaw

1 (15oz) can chickpeas, drained and rinsed

¼ cup chopped sun-dried tomatoes (not packed in oil)

Pre-chopped veggies are one of the greatest modern conveniences because they save so much time and enable you to enjoy more of the healthiest foods on the planet. Broccoli slaw is a perfect example, and it is now easy to find in almost every market. Loaded with huge doses of phytonutrition and scant on calories, broccoli slaw is the perfect toss-in-a-bowl ingredient. We added some hearty chickpeas, savory sun-dried tomatoes, and a lovely light and creamy tahini dressing to top it off.

1   In a blender, combine the tahini, lemon juice, garlic, tamari, black pepper, and 6 tablespoons warm water. Blend until smooth and well combined.

2   In a large bowl, combine the broccoli slaw, chickpeas, and sun-dried tomatoes. Pour in the dressing and toss to combine. Serve immediately or store in the refrigerator (with dressing stored separately) for up to 4 days.

✎   NOTE: For a slightly sweeter and more nuanced flavor, replace 1½ teaspoons lemon juice with 2 teaspoons balsamic.

COLESLAW

PREP TIME: **10 MINUTES**
COOK TIME: **NONE**
YIELD: **4 CUPS**

INGREDIENTS

4 cups coleslaw mix or equal parts
  shredded white cabbage, purple
  cabbage, and carrots

¼ cup **Mayonnaise** (page 241)

2 tsp apple cider vinegar

1 tsp maple syrup

½ tsp freshly squeezed lemon juice

¼ tsp freshly ground black pepper

Classically crunchy, creamy, and comforting, nothing feels more "summer in the USA" than a hefty helping of fresh coleslaw. Combining silky smooth mayo with ample veggie shreds, this simple salad is a staple that can be enjoyed at any time of the year.

1   Place the coleslaw mix in a large serving dish. Mix in the mayonnaise, apple cider vinegar, maple syrup, lemon juice, and black pepper, and toss to combine.

2   Serve immediately with the Deep South Bowl (page 150) or on its own, or store in an airtight container in the refrigerator for up to 4 days.

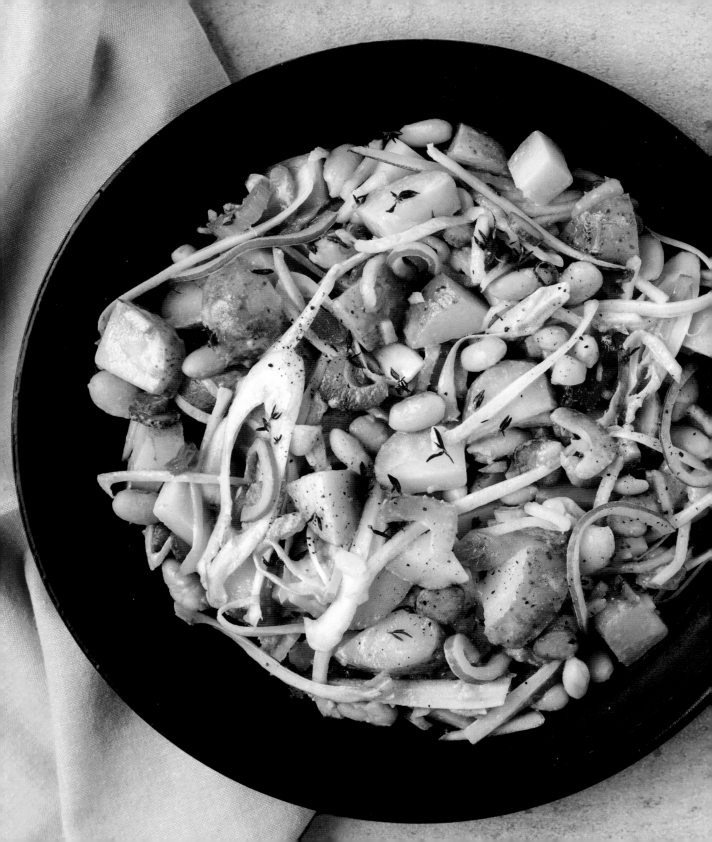

CAPE COD APPLE-CANNELLINI BEAN SALAD

PREP TIME: **30 MINUTES**
COOK TIME: **10 MINUTES**
YIELD: **2 SERVINGS**

INGREDIENTS

½ cup thinly sliced red or Vidalia onion

½ cup seasoned rice vinegar (just enough to cover onions)

1½ cups diced Yukon Gold potatoes (about ½lb total)

1 (15oz) can white cannellini beans, drained and rinsed

1 cup shaved endive leaves

1½ cups julienned green apple

½ cup thinly sliced celery

7 cornichons, thinly sliced

¼ cup golden raisins

1 tbsp fresh thyme, de-stemmed

2 tbsp freshly squeezed lemon juice

2 tsp olive oil

2 tsp Dijon mustard

Freshly ground black pepper, to taste

Ray discovered this perfectly balanced, unassuming salad at a restaurant in Cape Cod several years ago. He mastered his own version, impressing Julieanna with the satisfying flavors and textures, and it has become a regular treat that could happily be enjoyed on a weekly basis.

1 Place the sliced onions in a small bowl or airtight container. Add enough seasoned rice vinegar to cover the onions. Cover and place in the refrigerator to pickle for 30 minutes or more. (See note.)

2 Bring a large saucepan of water to a boil over medium-high heat. Once boiling, reduce the heat to a simmer and add the diced potatoes. Cook until fork-tender, about 10 minutes, and then drain.

3 In a large serving bowl, combine the potatoes, beans, endive, apple, celery, cornichons, raisins, and thyme.

4 In a small bowl, whisk together the lemon juice, olive oil, and mustard. Drizzle over the salad and toss to combine. Top with some pickled onions and sprinkle with black pepper. Enjoy immediately, or keep the salad in the refrigerator and allow the flavors to marinate further and enjoy the next day.

✎ **NOTE:** You can pickle the onions in seasoned rice vinegar in an airtight container in the refrigerator overnight. Pickled onions will last several days (or even weeks) and can be used as a topping on sandwiches, burritos, pizzas, salads, and more.

CHILI AVOCADO CITRUS BOWL

PREP TIME: 15 MINUTES
COOK TIME: NONE
YIELD: 1–2 SERVINGS

INGREDIENTS

2 medium oranges (see note),
  peeled and segmented or
  supremed, divided

1 tbsp seasoned rice vinegar

½ tsp chili powder

2 cups spring mix, sliced thin

1 grapefruit, peeled and segmented
  or supremed

½ cup chopped avocado

2 tbsp pomegranate arils

Citrusy freshness with a bit of a bite is the hallmark of this bowl. Subtle seasonings enhance the natural flavors of sour grapefruit and orange, tart pomegranate, and buttery avocado, which are topped off with a kick from chili powder and tossed over spring greens for a mouthwatering combination.

1   In a blender, combine segments from ½ orange, rice vinegar, and chili powder, and blend until smooth.

2   Place the spring mix, grapefruit segments, and remaining orange segments in a large serving bowl. Top with the avocado and pomegranate arils. Drizzle the dressing over the salad and serve immediately.

✎ **NOTE:** Replacing half of the oranges with blood oranges, when available, is a fantastic alternative.

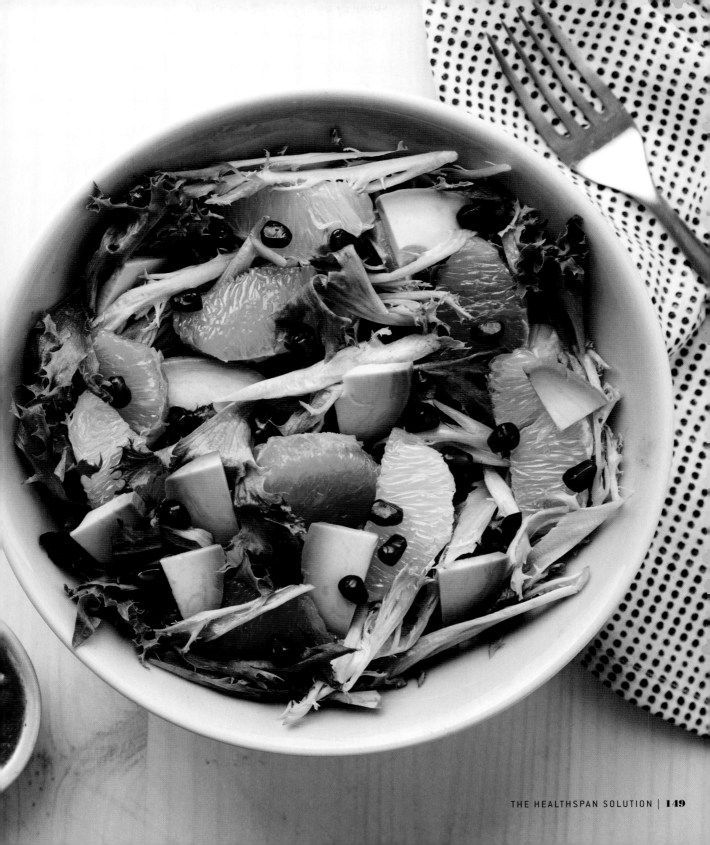

DEEP SOUTH BOWL
with Alabama White Sauce

PREP TIME: **10 MINUTES**
COOK TIME: **20 MINUTES**
YIELD: **2 SERVINGS**

INGREDIENTS

1 (15oz) can black-eyed peas, drained and rinsed

1 tsp hot sauce, such as Tabasco Original Red Sauce

¼ tsp liquid smoke

1 cup diced yellow onion

1 small yellow squash, quartered lengthwise and thickly sliced

1 small zucchini, quartered lengthwise and thickly sliced

¼ tsp garlic powder

1 tbsp apple cider vinegar

4 cups chopped collard greens, de-stemmed (3–4 collard leaves)

1 tsp molasses

1 (15oz) can stewed tomatoes and okra or 1 (15oz) can stewed tomatoes and 1 cup frozen okra

1 cup corn kernels

2 cups cooked brown rice, cooled

2 cups **Coleslaw** (page 145)

¼ cup **Alabama White Sauce** (page 240)

You won't find smoked chicken, pulled pork, or ribs in this book. But, truth be told, those are just excuses in Alabama to eat white sauce. So, here is our healthy, decadent, down-home Southern bowl loaded with all the fixins' that represent the local flavors and traditions…and we reckon it's a great excuse to whip up our version of North Alabama's famous sauce.

1   In a medium bowl, combine the black-eyed peas, hot sauce, and liquid smoke. Heat in the microwave or in a small saucepan until warmed. Set aside.

2   Heat a medium saucepan over medium-high heat. Dry sauté the onions until they begin to brown. Add the yellow squash, zucchini, and 1 tablespoon water. Cover and steam for 3 to 5 minutes. Add 1 teaspoon water to deglaze the pan, and sprinkle with garlic powder. Cover and cook for 2 minutes more until the water begins to evaporate. Transfer the vegetables to a dish and set aside.

3   Wipe out the saucepan and return to the burner over medium-high heat. Add ¼ cup water, apple cider vinegar, and collards. Cover and steam for 10 minutes until soft, but not wilted. Remove from the heat, drizzle with molasses, and mix. Set aside.

4   Heat a separate large saucepan over medium-high heat. Once hot, add the corn to the dry pan and roast until the kernels begin to brown, 4 to 5 minutes. Transfer the corn to the dish with the cooked vegetables and set aside.

5   Wipe out the saucepan used for the corn and heat over medium-high heat. Add the stewed tomatoes and okra. Bring to a boil. Lower the heat, cover, and simmer for 5 minutes. Remove from the heat.

6   To assemble, divide each component evenly between two large salad bowls. Each bowl should have about 1 cup cooked brown rice, ½ cup black-eyed peas, 1 cup squash, 1 cup collard greens, 1 cup Coleslaw, ½ cup stewed tomatoes with okra, and ½ cup roasted corn. Top each bowl with 2 tablespoons Alabama White Sauce and enjoy immediately.

✎ **NOTE:** This bowl is quick to throw together when using batch-cooked or frozen brown rice and corn, pre-chopped veggies, and Alabama White Sauce (page 240) and Mayonnaise (page 241)—both of which can happily maintain regular real estate in the refrigerator. You can double or triple each of these recipes and enjoy your Deep South Bowl throughout the week.

FAJITA SALAD
with Mango Roasted Corn Salsa

PREP TIME: **20 MINUTES**
COOK TIME: **10 MINUTES**
YIELD: **2 SERVINGS**

INGREDIENTS

1½ cups sliced green bell pepper

1½ cups sliced red bell pepper

1½ cups sliced yellow onion

1½ cups sliced red onion

2 medium Portobello mushroom caps, sliced

½ cup pickled jalapeños, diced

2 tbsp freshly squeezed lime juice

2 cups chopped romaine and iceberg lettuce

½ cup julienned jicama

1 cup **Mango Roasted Corn Salsa** (page 203)

¼ avocado, thinly sliced

For the seasoning

1 tsp chili powder

1 tsp paprika

1 tsp garlic powder

½ tsp onion powder

½ tsp ground cumin

½ tsp dried oregano

¼ tsp freshly ground black pepper

For the dressing

¼ cup sun-dried tomatoes (not in oil)

2 tbsp ketchup

2 tbsp freshly squeezed lime juice

1 tsp chili powder

¼ cup unsweetened nondairy milk

Have you ever gone out for Mexican food and been torn between a tostada and the fajitas? Between crisp, fresh, and cool and hot, sizzling, and hearty? Well, this salad is a combination of the two, encompassing all the deliciousness, so you don't have to choose. Topped with our mouthwatering Mango Roasted Corn Salsa (which could easily be eaten on its own) and an umami-rich dressing, we love this happy hybrid.

1 In a small bowl, combine all seasoning ingredients and mix well. Set aside.

2 In a blender, combine all dressing ingredients along with ¼ cup warm water and blend until smooth. Set aside.

3 Heat a large wok or sauté pan over medium-high heat. Add the bell peppers, onions, and mushroom slices to the pan along with 2 tablespoons water. Cover and steam for 1 to 2 minutes. Remove the lid and cook for 7 to 8 minutes or until the vegetables are browned. Stir in the fajita seasoning, jalapeños, and lime juice. Cook until the liquid is fully absorbed.

4 Place the lettuce and jicama in a large serving bowl. Top with the fajita vegetables, Mango Roasted Corn Salsa, and avocado. Drizzle with the dressing and serve immediately.

EAT YOUR GREENS BOWL

with Carrot-Ginger Dressing

PREP TIME: **15 MINUTES**
COOK TIME: **10 MINUTES**
YIELD: **2 SERVINGS**

INGREDIENTS

8–10 asparagus spears

4 cups chopped kale, de-stemmed

½ tsp low-sodium tamari

¼ tsp garlic powder

1 cup broccoli florets

Freshly squeezed lime juice,
  to taste

2 cups cooked brown rice

1 cup cooked shelled edamame

1 cup sliced English (hothouse)
  cucumber

½ avocado, cut into chunks

¼ cup fresh broccoli sprouts or
  microgreens

2 tsp hempseeds , to garnish

2 tbsp nori flakes, to garnish

For the dressing

¼ cup hempseeds

2 tbsp chopped fresh ginger

2 tbsp freshly squeezed lime juice

1 tbsp seasoned rice vinegar

½ tsp sesame oil

½ tsp white miso paste

1 tsp maple syrup

1 cup sliced carrots

How green is your bowl? Ray has his Deep South Bowl with Alabama White Sauce, so this California-style gorgeously green bowl (with hemp and sprouts for full effect) evens the playing field for the authors' bicoastal traditional roots.

1   Place the asparagus in a covered glass dish with 1 tablespoon water. Heat in the microwave until tender but still crisp. Set aside.

2   Heat a medium saucepan over medium-high heat. Add the kale, cover, and cook with 2 tablespoons water for 4 to 6 minutes, until wilted. Add the tamari and garlic powder, toss to combine, remove from the heat, and set aside.

3   Place the broccoli in a covered glass bowl or dish. Heat in the microwave until bright green and tender but still crisp. Squeeze lime juice over the broccoli and set aside.

4   To make the dressing, pulse ¼ cup hempseeds in a blender until ground to a powder but not a paste, approximately 30 seconds. Add the remaining dressing ingredients along with 2 tablespoons water and blend until smooth.

5   To assemble, divide the components evenly between two large salad bowls. Each bowl should have about 1 cup brown rice, 4 to 5 asparagus spears, 1 cup steamed kale, ½ cup steamed broccoli, ½ cup edamame, ½ cup cucumber, ¼ avocado, and 2 tablespoons sprouts. Drizzle each bowl with dressing, garnish with hempseeds and nori flakes, and enjoy immediately.

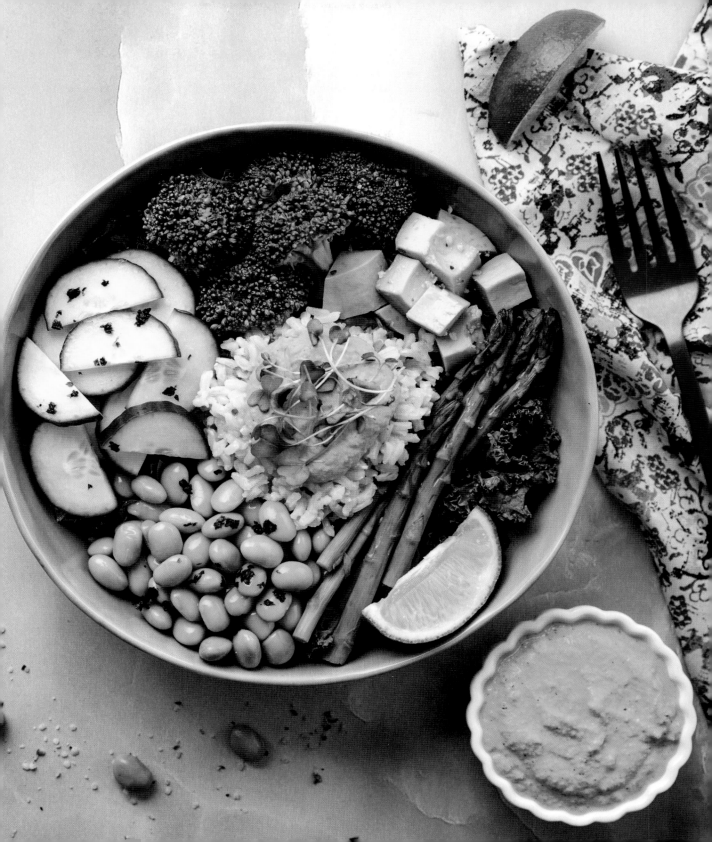

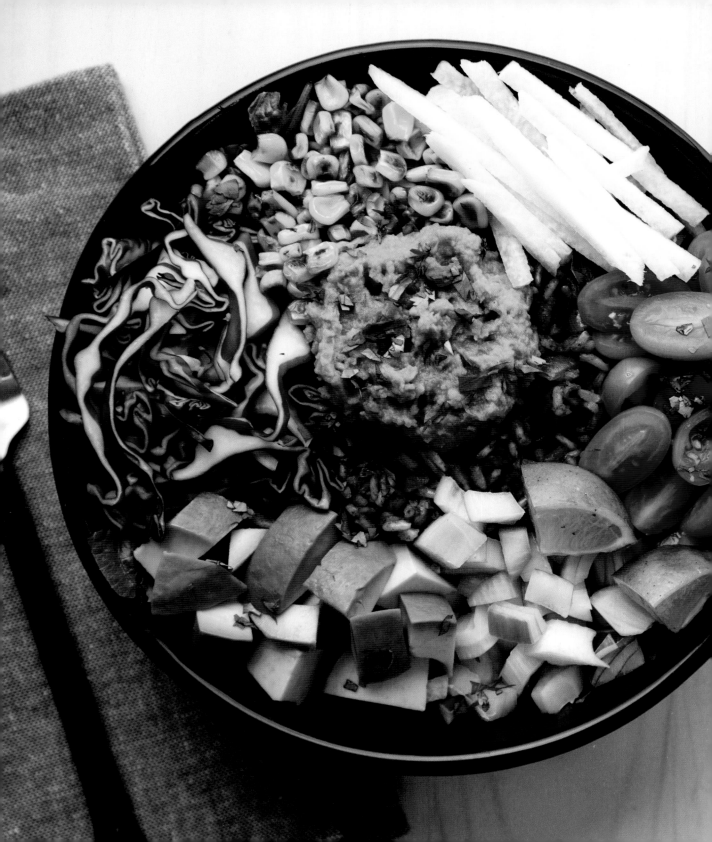

MEXICAN RICE BURRITO BOWL

PREP TIME: **15 MINUTES**
COOK TIME: **5 MINUTES**
YIELD: **4 SERVINGS**

INGREDIENTS

1 cup corn kernels, fresh or frozen

1 (15oz) can fat-free refried beans

1 tsp chipotle hot sauce, such as Tabasco Chipotle Pepper Sauce

8 cups chopped romaine lettuce

1 batch **Mexican Rice** (page 191)

2 cups chopped red cabbage

2 cups halved cherry tomatoes

1 cup julienned jicama

1 cup chopped avocado

½ cup chopped red onion

¼ cup minced cilantro, to garnish

Green chili habanero sauce, to serve

Lime wedges, to serve

Amigos, gear up for a fun fiesta in a bowl! With a collection of crunch and color, creamy refried beans, chewy Mexican Rice, sweet roasted corn, and hearty hints of heat, you can celebrate the flavors of Mexican cuisine with this *plato delicioso*.

1   Heat a large saucepan over medium-high heat. Once hot, add the corn and toast for about 5 minutes, until the kernels start to pop and are browned, stirring occasionally.

2   In a separate saucepan, heat the refried beans and hot sauce over medium heat, stirring frequently, for 3 to 5 minutes or until warm.

3   To build each bowl, begin with a bed of lettuce and top with 1 cup Mexican Rice and ⅓ cup refried beans. Add equal amounts of the roasted corn, red cabbage, tomatoes, jicama, avocado, and onions to each bowl. Garnish to taste with cilantro, habanero sauce, and lime.

✎ **NOTE:** The refried beans can be heated in the microwave, if desired.

QUINOA TABBOULEH SALAD
with Roasted Garlic and Pine Nut Dressing

PREP TIME: **15 MINUTES**
COOK TIME: **15 MINUTES**
YIELD: **2 SERVINGS**

INGREDIENTS

½ cup uncooked quinoa, rinsed

½ cup chopped cucumber

½ cup quartered grape or cherry tomatoes

¼ cup minced red onion

¼ cup chopped scallions

¼ cup minced fresh mint

¼ cup minced fresh Italian (flat-leaf) parsley

1 tbsp freshly squeezed lemon juice

1 tbsp low-sodium tamari

4 cups chopped romaine lettuce

1 tsp pine nuts, to garnish

For the dressing

¼ cup pine nuts

2 cloves roasted garlic (see note)

1 tbsp low-sodium tamari

1 tsp balsamic vinegar

1 tbsp freshly squeezed lemon juice

Originally from the Middle East, tabbouleh is a lightly seasoned salad traditionally made with finely chopped fresh herbs, tomato, and bulgur or couscous. This version uses nutrient-dense quinoa as the base and is dressed in a savory, garlicky sauce.

1   In a small saucepan, the combine quinoa and 1 cup water and bring to a boil over medium-high heat. Lower the heat, cover, and simmer for 10 to 15 minutes, until all the water is absorbed. Once the water is absorbed, remove from heat, keep covered, and allow to steam for 5 minutes. Fluff with a fork and transfer to a large bowl.

2   To the bowl with the quinoa, add the cucumber, tomatoes, onions, scallions, mint, parsley, lemon juice, and tamari. Toss well to combine.

3   To make the dressing, in a blender, pulse the pine nuts to a fine powder. Add the roasted garlic, tamari, balsamic vinegar, lemon juice, and 1 tablespoon warm water. Blend until well combined and smooth.

4   Divide the lettuce evenly between two bowls. Top each bowl with the quinoa mixture, drizzle with dressing, and sprinkle with pine nuts. Serve immediately.

✎ **NOTES:** Roasted garlic is a great ingredient to have on hand to boost flavors in recipes. Typically, roasting involves coating the garlic with oil to prevent oxidation during the cooking process, protect the surface from drying, and encourage browning. To create a similar flavor without the oil, cut the top off the garlic bulb. Place the garlic bulb root-side up (cut-side-down) in a muffin pan to slow down or reduce access to the air while cooking. Roast at 400°F for 30 to 40 minutes.

Roasted garlic can be stored in an airtight container in the refrigerator for 3 to 4 days or in the freezer for up to a year. To freeze, remove the papery shell and separate the garlic cloves. Place the roasted garlic in an empty ice cube tray and freeze for 1 hour. Once frozen, toss them in a freezer bag, and these individual cloves will last up to a year.

HERBED DIJON POTATO SALAD

PREP TIME: **20 MINUTES**
COOK TIME: **15 MINUTES**
YIELD: **4–6 SERVINGS**

INGREDIENTS

1lb red fingerling potatoes, quartered

1lb yellow fingerling potatoes, quartered

$\frac{1}{3}$ cup diced carrots

$\frac{1}{3}$ cup diced celery

$\frac{1}{3}$ cup diced yellow onion

4 scallions, thinly sliced

$\frac{1}{4}$ cup minced fresh dill

$\frac{1}{4}$ cup flat-leaf (Italian) parsley, de-stemmed and minced

For the dressing

1 cup hempseeds

3 garlic cloves, minced

2 tbsp apple cider vinegar

2 tbsp Dijon mustard

1 tbsp maple syrup or molasses

1 tbsp low-sodium tamari

1 tsp chipotle hot sauce, such as Tabasco Chipotle Pepper Sauce

$\frac{1}{4}$ tsp freshly ground black pepper

We love potatoes! Considered one of the most satiating foods because of their starch, fiber, and water content, they also happen to be rich in micronutrients, such as potassium and vitamins B6 and C. Fun fact: a baked potato, gram for gram, has a better amino acid score than 90-percent lean beef! This salad is herbaceous, fragrant, and creamy, and it is the perfect picnic-friendly side dish.

1   Place the potatoes in a pot or large saucepan and add enough water to cover by about 2 inches. Bring to a boil over medium-high heat. Reduce the heat to low and simmer for 10 to 15 minutes or until the potatoes can be easily pierced with a fork. Drain and set aside to cool.

2   In a blender, combine all dressing ingredients along with ½ cup water and blend for 60 to 90 seconds or until smooth. Add more water if needed to reach your desired consistency.

3   In a large serving bowl, place the cooled potatoes, carrots, celery, onions, scallions, dill, and parsley. Pour the dressing over the mixture and toss to combine. Serve warm immediately or refrigerate to allow the flavors to marinate, and serve cold.

APPLE SPINACH SALAD
with Orange-Rosemary Dressing

PREP TIME: **15 MINUTES**
COOK TIME: **NONE**
YIELD: **1 SERVING**

INGREDIENTS

2–3 cups baby spinach leaves, rolled and sliced

1 medium Granny Smith apple, cut into matchsticks

1 medium Jazz or Honeycrisp apple, cut into matchsticks

1–2 tbsp minced red onion

For the dressing

2 tsp minced fresh rosemary

1 small orange, peeled and segmented

1 garlic clove

1 tsp anchovy-free Worcestershire sauce

Steeping herbs to make an infusion is a subtle way to add depth of flavor to a dish. Pungently piney rosemary pairs perfectly with bright, zesty orange and is rounded off with garlic and Worcestershire sauce to spruce up these staple salad ingredients.

1. Place the rosemary in a small bowl and add 2 tablespoons hot water. Let stand for 2 to 3 minutes to infuse.

2. Transfer the rosemary-infused water (with leaves) to a blender and add the orange segments (be sure to remove any seeds), garlic, and Worcestershire sauce. Blend until smooth.

3. Place the spinach, apples, and onions in a serving bowl. Pour the dressing over the salad and serve immediately.

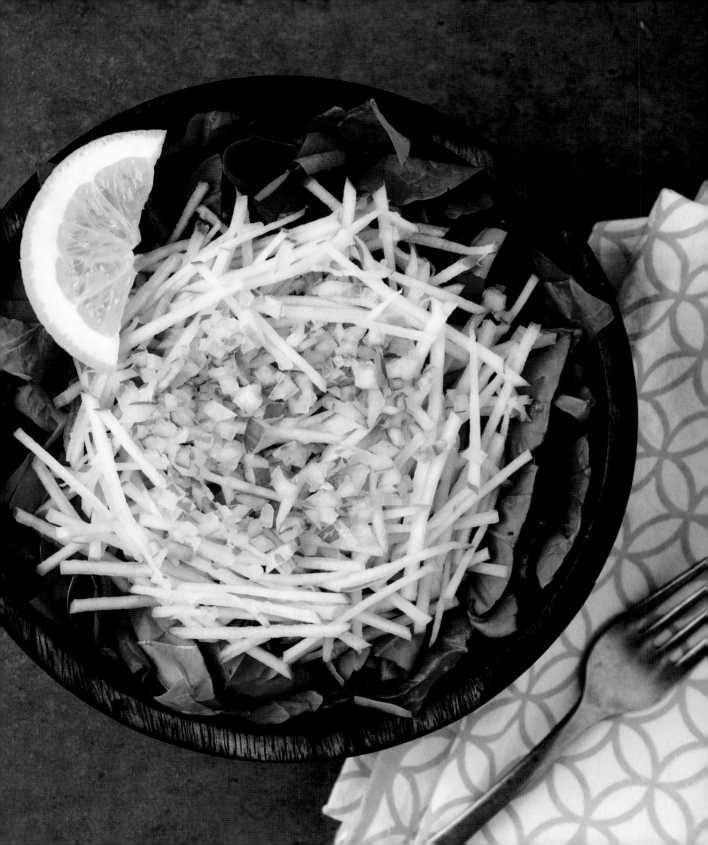

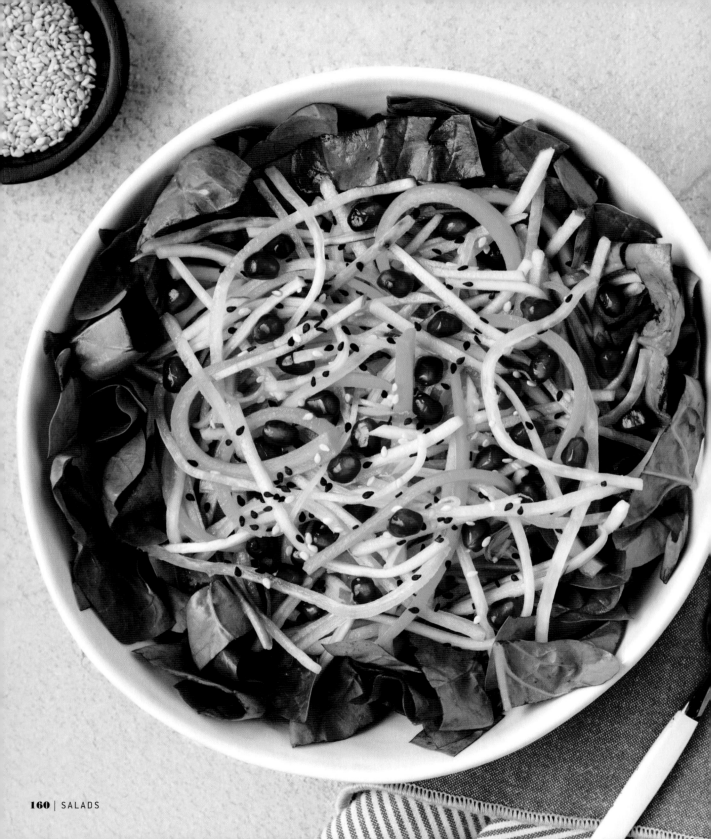

DAIKON, CUCUMBER, AND APPLE SALAD

with Sesame Dressing

PREP TIME: **30 MINUTES**
COOK TIME: **NONE**
YIELD: **2 SERVINGS**

INGREDIENTS

¼ large (3-in diameter) daikon radish

1 English (hothouse) cucumber

5 small carrots

2 medium crisp red apples, such as Honeycrisp, Jazz, or Pink Lady

3 cups chopped baby spinach

½ cup pomegranate arils

For the dressing

1 tbsp seasoned rice wine vinegar

½ tsp low-sodium tamari

½ tsp sesame oil

To garnish (optional)

2 tbsp sliced scallions

½ tsp black sesame seeds

½ tsp toasted sesame seeds

Squeeze of lime

Sriracha

Daikon, "long root," is a mild winter radish perhaps most commonly used as a garnish for sushi and sashimi dishes at Japanese restaurants. This cruciferous veggie tastes like crunchy water with a mildly bitter, "radishy" undertone, and is bursting with healthy nutrition. Together with cool cucumbers, sweet carrots and apples, tart pomegranates, and simple seasonings, this salad is scrumptious.

1. Using a mandoline slicer or a knife, cut the daikon radish, cucumber, carrots, and apples into matchstick slices.

2. To make the dressing, in a small bowl, whisk together the rice vinegar, tamari, and sesame oil.

3. Divide the spinach evenly between two salad bowls and layer the radish, cucumber, carrots, and apples on top. Add the pomegranate arils and drizzle with dressing. Top with additional garnishes, as desired, and serve immediately.

ROASTED CAULIFLOWER SALAD
with Sweet Dijon Dressing

PREP TIME: **10 MINUTES**
COOK TIME: **25 MINUTES**
YIELD: **4–6 SERVINGS**

INGREDIENTS

1 medium head cauliflower, any color, cut into florets (about 4 cups)

1½ cups baby spinach

1½ cups arugula

¼ cup golden raisins

1 tbsp sliced almonds

Freshly squeezed lemon juice (optional), to taste

For the dressing

¼ cup raw cashews

1 tbsp apple cider vinegar

1 tbsp sliced scallions, white and light green parts only

1 tbsp raisins or 1 Medjool date

2 tsp Dijon mustard

1 tsp low-sodium tamari

¼ tsp freshly ground black pepper

½ cup unsweetened nondairy milk

Roasting cauliflower magnifies its magnificence, bringing out its sweetness and softening its fibers, turning it into something extra special. In this salad, we made this top-Triangle cruciferous food the centerpiece, plating it over greens and topping it with a sprinkle of raisins and almonds and a drizzle of sweet dijon dressing.

1   Preheat oven to 425°F and line a baking sheet with a silicone baking mat or parchment paper.

2   Spread the cauliflower in an even layer on the prepared pan and roast for 20 to 25 minutes, until tender and edges are golden brown.

3   In a blender, pulse the cashews to a fine powder, but not all the way to a paste. Add the remaining dressing ingredients and blend until smooth.

4   Place the baby spinach and arugula in a large serving bowl. Top with the roasted cauliflower, golden raisins, and almonds. Drizzle with dressing and a splash of lemon juice, if desired. Enjoy immediately.

PORTOBELLO MUSHROOM CAESAR
with Avocado and Sun-Dried Tomatoes

PREP TIME: **20 MINUTES**
COOK TIME: **10 MINUTES**
YIELD: **2 SERVINGS**

INGREDIENTS

2 medium Portobello mushroom caps, sliced

1 (15oz) can butter beans, drained and rinsed

½ cup sun-dried tomatoes (not packed in oil)

2 tbsp balsamic vinegar

6 cups chopped romaine lettuce

2 slices sprouted whole grain bread, cut into small squares and toasted to make croutons

½ avocado, chopped

For the dressing

⅓ cup raw cashews

2 tbsp nutritional yeast

2 garlic-stuffed green olives, rinsed (or 1 tbsp drained black olive slices)

1 tsp capers, drained

2 tsp anchovy-free Worcestershire sauce

2 tsp Dijon mustard

2 tbsp lemon juice

¼ cup unsweetened nondairy milk

1 garlic clove

¾ tsp freshly ground black pepper

1 tsp nori flakes

Caesar salads are classically focused on the crisp lettuce, crunchy croutons, and a creamy, briny dressing. We swapped in capers and olives for brine and nori for a mild fish flavor along with silky butter beans, hearty mushrooms, and crisp lettuce for a plant-based version that doesn't disappoint.

1 To make the dressing, in a blender, blend the cashews and nutritional yeast until a fine powder forms, about 30 seconds. Add the remaining dressing ingredients, blend until smooth, and set aside.

2 Heat a saucepan over medium-high heat. Add the mushrooms and cook for about 5 minutes until their liquid is released. Add the butter beans, sun-dried tomatoes, and vinegar and cook for 2 to 3 minutes, until the balsamic is reduced down, but not dry. Remove from heat.

3 Divide the lettuce evenly between two large salad bowls. Drizzle with dressing and toss. Top with the mushroom mix, croutons, and avocado. Enjoy immediately.

BBQ CHICKPEA CHOPPED SALAD
with Creamy Southwest Dressing

PREP TIME: **10 MINUTES**
COOK TIME: **10 MINUTES**
YIELD: **2 SERVINGS**

INGREDIENTS

1 (15oz) can low-sodium chickpeas, drained and rinsed

½ cup diced red onion

3 tbsp **Easy Homemade Barbecue Sauce** (page 240) or store-bought BBQ sauce

2 ears of corn (see note)

1 tsp smoked paprika

2 cups chopped romaine or butter lettuce

½ cup chopped jicama (see note)

½ cup halved cherry or grape tomatoes

½ cup chopped avocado

For the dressing

¼ cup raw cashews

1 tbsp **Easy Homemade Barbecue Sauce** (page 240) or store-bought BBQ sauce

2 tsp apple cider vinegar

½ tsp onion powder

¼ cup + 1 tbsp unsweetened nondairy milk

¼ tsp dried dill

Tangy, skillet-warmed chickpeas; sweet, smoky corn; ample crunch; and flavors of the Southwest make this recipe a perfect weekday meal to quickly throw together and satisfy your craving for barbecue.

1   In a medium skillet over medium-high heat, add the chickpeas and onions, and cook until the onions are translucent and the chickpeas are dry, 3 to 5 minutes. Pour the Barbecue Sauce over the chickpeas and onions and toss to combine. Remove from heat and set aside.

2   Place the corn ears, with husks, in the microwave and heat for 5 minutes. Remove from the microwave. Using a pot holder to grip the husk, cut off the base, just beyond the curve, and shake the corn ear out of the husk. Cut the corn kernels off the cob and place in a bowl. Add the smoked paprika, toss to combine, and set aside.

3   Make the dressing. In a blender, pulse the cashews to a fine powder, but stop before they form a paste. Add all the remaining dressing ingredients and blend until smooth and well combined.

4   Divide the lettuce evenly between two salad bowls and top with the chickpeas, corn, jicama, tomatoes, and avocado. Drizzle the dressing over each salad. Serve immediately.

✎ **NOTES:** If fresh corn is unavailable, you can use 1 cup defrosted frozen corn kernels.

For ease of peeling, slice off the ends of the jicama first.

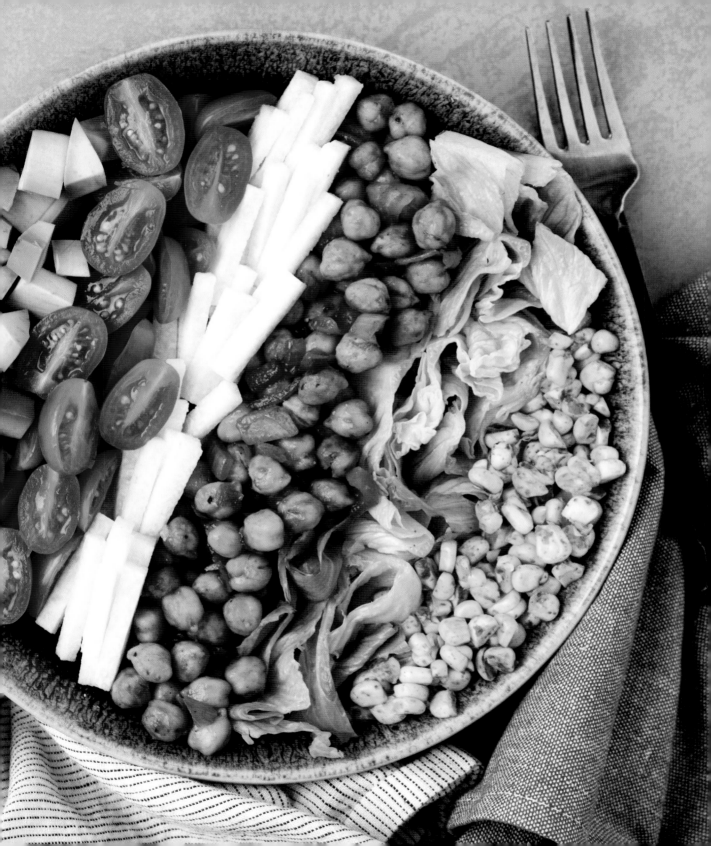

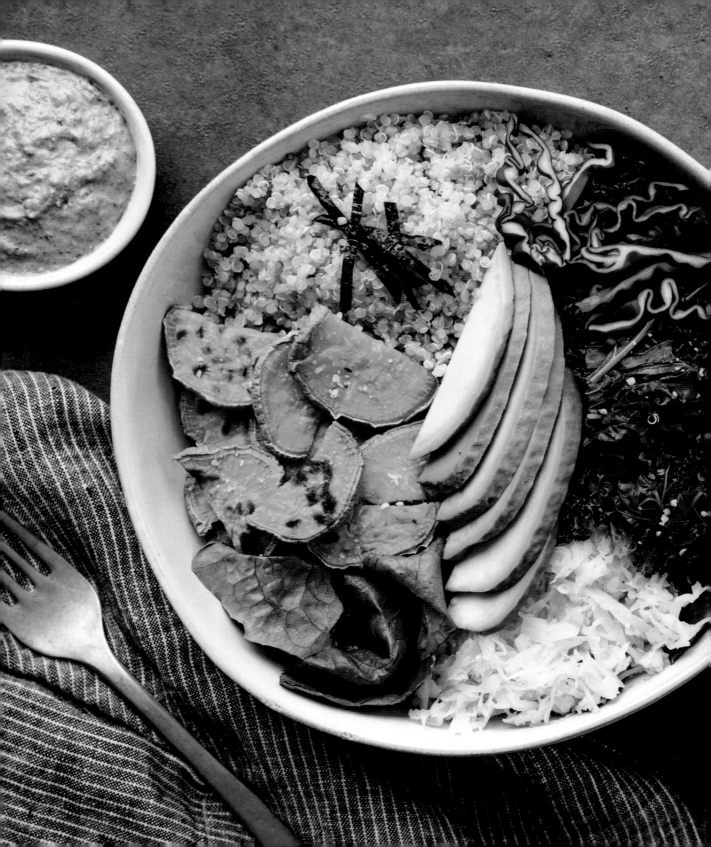

FLOURISH BOWL
with Green Goddess Dressing

PREP TIME: **10 MINUTES**
COOK TIME: **40 MINUTES**
YIELD: **2 SERVINGS**

INGREDIENTS

1 small sweet potato

½ cup uncooked quinoa, rinsed

3 cups chopped kale

6 cups chopped romaine lettuce

½ avocado, sliced

½ cup thinly sliced red cabbage

½ cup sauerkraut

2 tbsp nori strips or nori sprinkles

2 tsp hempseeds

For the dressing

1 cup chopped fresh chives

1 cup chopped fresh parsley

2 garlic cloves

4 tbsp tahini

4 tbsp nutritional yeast

2 tbsp miso paste

4 tbsp freshly squeezed lemon juice

1 tbsp chia seeds

"Flourish" means to grow, thrive, and prosper. Placing a little bit of every nutritious food (vegetables, fruits, whole grains, legumes, mushrooms, nuts, seeds, herbs, and spices) into one fantastic bowl is a recipe for flourishing. This bowl is quick to whip up and even easier if you keep batches of quinoa and the Green Goddess Dressing (fantastic on any salad) ready to go in your refrigerator.

1 Preheat the oven to 400°F and line a baking sheet with a silicone baking mat or parchment paper. Slice the unpeeled sweet potato into ½-inch-thick rounds and spread evenly on the prepared pan. Bake for 40 minutes, flipping halfway through.

2 Meanwhile, in a medium saucepan, combine the quinoa and 1 cup water. Bring to a boil over medium-high heat. Once boiling, reduce the heat to low, cover, and cook for 10 to 15 minutes until all the water is absorbed. Remove from the heat to cool for 5 minutes and then fluff with a fork.

3 Heat a large wok or saucepan over medium-high heat. Add the kale and 2 tablespoons water. Cover to steam for 4 to 6 minutes. Set aside.

4 To make the dressing, in a blender, combine the chives, parsley, and garlic and blend for a few seconds. Add the tahini, nutritional yeast, miso paste, lemon juice, chia seeds, and ⅔ cup water. Blend until smooth.

5 Divide the lettuce evenly between two salad bowls. To each bowl, add half the cooked quinoa, sweet potato rounds, and steamed kale. Top each bowl with avocado, cabbage, sauerkraut, nori, and hempseeds. Drizzle the dressing over top and enjoy immediately.

NOTE: To save time, keep items such as sweet potatoes, grains, and a good dressing prepped and ready to go for the week. You can quickly toss them together in varying combinations for quick, wholesome, and satisfying meals.

SPICY SOUTHWEST SALAD
with Smoky Red Pepper Dressing

PREP TIME: **20 MINUTES**
COOK TIME: **5 MINUTES**
YIELD: **2 SERVINGS**

INGREDIENTS

2 romaine hearts, chopped

4 cups cruciferous greens mix

½ cup thinly sliced red onion

1 red bell pepper, diced (reserve top and bottom ends for dressing)

10–12 pickled jalapeño peppers

For the dressing

¼ cup raw cashews

3 tbsp nutritional yeast

¼ tsp cayenne

½ tsp hot smoked paprika

1 red bell pepper, top (stem removed) and bottom only

3 tbsp ketchup

2 tbsp freshly squeezed lime juice

½ cup unsweetened nondairy milk

For the topping

1 cup corn kernels, fresh or frozen

1 tsp chili powder

½ tsp chipotle powder

1 cup canned black beans

This is one of our most repeated recipes at home, because it combines our much-beloved flavors and textures. The contrast of the crisp and fresh greens, bell peppers, and onions with the warm and spicy beans and corn makes this salad simply spectacular.

1   Divide the lettuce, cruciferous greens mix, and red onions evenly between two large salad bowls. (If you don't enjoy the flavor of raw onions, they can be cooked with the corn in step 3.)

2   To prepare the dressing, in a food processor, pulse the cashews, nutritional yeast, cayenne, and smoked paprika until a fine powder forms. (Stop before the mixture turns into a paste.) Add the bell pepper ends, ketchup, lime juice, and nondairy milk and blend until smooth and creamy. If the consistency is too thick, add additional nondairy milk, 1 tablespoon at a time.

3   To prepare the topping, in a dry nonstick pan, roast the corn over medium-high heat for 3 to 5 minutes, until it begins to caramelize. It should have brown or blackish spots, but try not to scorch it too much. (If you prefer to sauté the onion rather than eating it raw, add it to the corn.)

4   Stir in the chili powder and chipotle powder. Add the black beans with a little of the liquid from the can. Cook for 1 to 2 minutes, just long enough to heat the beans.

5   Drizzle the dressing over the greens, dividing it evenly between the two bowls. Top each bowl with an equal portion of the hot corn and bean mixture, and then add the diced bell pepper and jalapeño slices.

SPINACH BERRY SALAD
with Poppy Seed Dressing

PREP TIME: **10 MINUTES**
COOK TIME: **NONE**
YIELD: **2 SERVINGS**

INGREDIENTS

3 cups baby spinach, roughly
  chopped
½ cup blueberries
½ cup sliced strawberries
4 tbsp sliced almonds

For the dressing

1 tbsp chia seeds
¼ cup unsweetened nondairy milk
1 tbsp + ½ tsp apple cider vinegar
1 cup green grapes
1½ tsp Dijon mustard
2 tsp poppy seeds

We both grew up loving a classic spinach salad with poppy seed dressing. Using white grapes to sweeten and chia seeds to thicken, this lovely version is made with healthspan-centered ingredients.

1 To make the dressing, in a blender, pulse the chia seeds into a powder. Add the nondairy milk, vinegar, grapes, mustard, and 2 tablespoons water and blend until smooth. Add the poppy seeds and stir to combine.

2 Divide the spinach evenly between 2 salad bowls. To each bowl, add an equal amount of blueberries, strawberries, and almonds. Drizzle dressing over each salad and serve immediately.

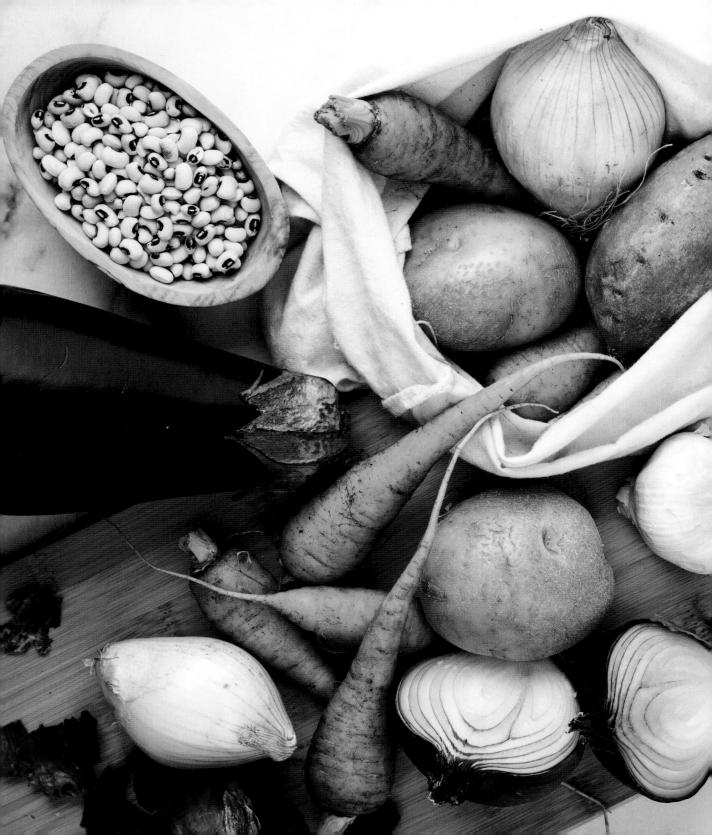

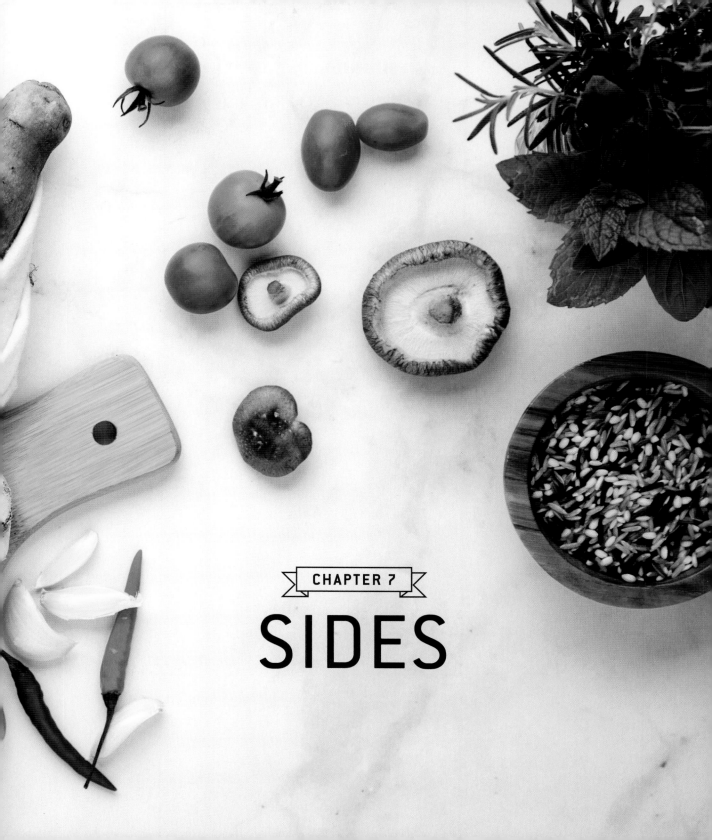

CHAPTER 7

SIDES

TACO CASSEROLE

PREP TIME: **15 MINUTES**
COOK TIME: **45 MINUTES**
YIELD: **4–6 SERVINGS**

INGREDIENTS

1 (15oz) can low-sodium black beans, drained and rinsed

1 (15oz) can low-sodium pinto beans, drained and rinsed

1 tbsp chili powder

1 tsp ground cumin

½ tsp garlic powder

½ tsp onion powder

½ tsp dried Mexican oregano

½ tsp smoked paprika

1 (15oz) can fire-roasted tomatoes

1 tbsp cornstarch

½ cup corn kernels

½ cup diced red onion

½ cup diced red bell pepper

½ cup diced green bell pepper

12 corn tortillas, cut into quarters

1 batch **Chipotle Butternut Cheesy Sauce** (page 239)

½ cup sliced scallions

Serve taco night in an easy baked dish, with a layered casserole of corn tortillas, piquant velvety beans, sweet roasted corn, and smoky butternut "cheese." Delve into this deconstructed taco with a side of avocado or guacamole and salsa to top off this full comfort-food experience.

1   Preheat the oven to 375°F. In a food processor, pulse the black beans and pinto beans until smooth. Transfer to a large bowl and stir in the chili powder, cumin, garlic powder, onion powder, oregano, and paprika.

2   In a separate medium bowl, combine the tomatoes and cornstarch, stir, and set aside.

3   Heat a large saucepan over medium-high heat. Once hot, add the corn and dry pan-roast until it begins to brown, approximately 4 to 5 minutes. Add the onions and continue dry sauté for an additional 1 to 2 minutes. Add the bell peppers and continue cooking until the vegetables soften, 3 to 5 minutes. Add 1 tablespoon water to deglaze the pan and stir. Remove from the heat.

4   In a 9 × 9-inch glass or ceramic casserole dish, layer a third of the tortilla triangles (4 tortillas) on the bottom. Spread with half of the bean mixture followed by half of the vegetable mix and half of the tomatoes. Repeat with another layer of tortilla triangles (4 tortillas), the remaining beans, and the remaining vegetables. Top with the remaining tomatoes and a final layer of tortilla triangles (4 tortillas).

5   Cover with aluminum foil and bake 20 minutes. Remove foil and bake 10 minutes more.

6   Remove from the oven, spoon the Chipotle Butternut Cheesy Sauce over the top, sprinkle with the scallions, and enjoy.

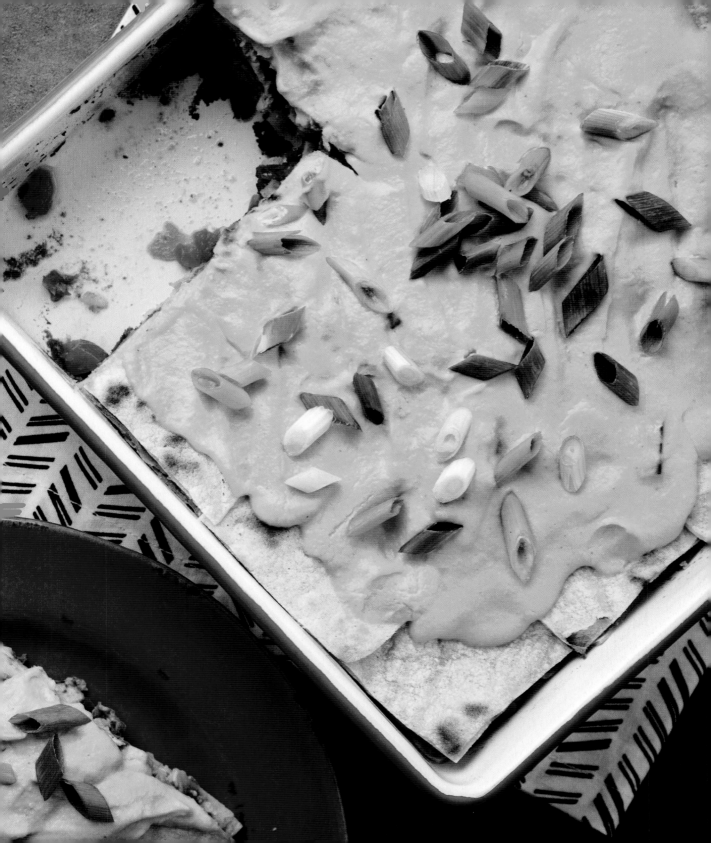

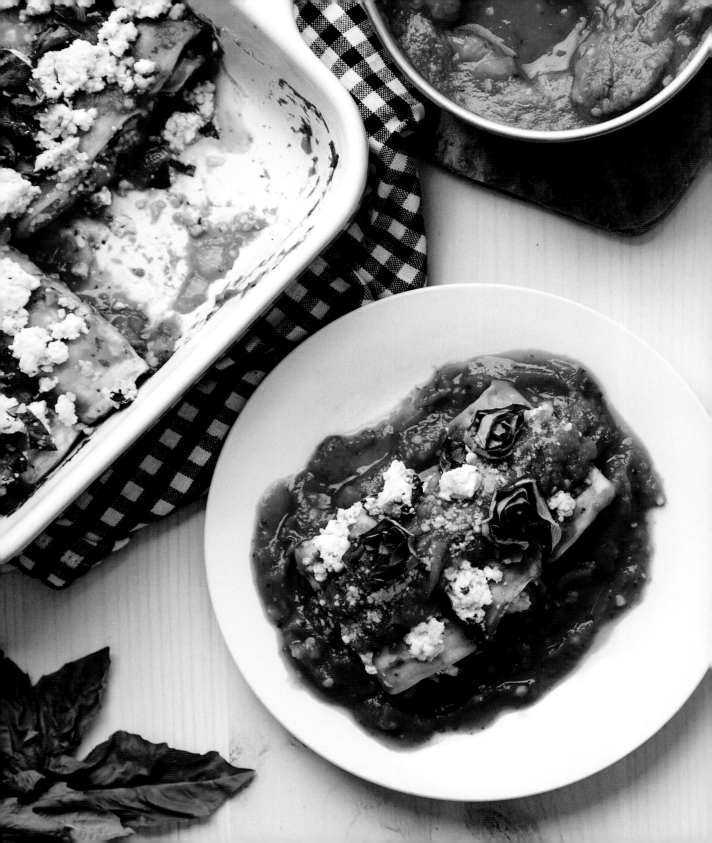

EGGPLANT ROLLATINI

PREP TIME: **15 MINUTES**
COOK TIME: **1 HOUR 5 MINUTES**
YIELD: **6 SERVINGS**

INGREDIENTS

3 large eggplants (to make about 28 ¼-in slices)

2–3 cups finely chopped kale

1 batch **Tofu Ricotta** (page 238)

4–6 cups **Grandma Marie's Tomato Sauce** (page 241)

To garnish

2 tbsp basil chiffonade

Crushed red pepper flakes

Cashew Parmesan Sprinkle (page 239)

Comfort food? Check! Soft, tangy, plant-based ricotta cheese is wrapped in tender eggplant, covered in warm umami-rich tomato sauce, and topped with a delicate basil chiffonade for a people-pleasing recipe offering decadence at its finest. It's amazing hot out of the oven, or let the flavors meld while it waits to be tomorrow's leftovers in the fridge. (That is, if there's any left to put in the fridge.) This dish, especially when prepared with our Grandma Marie's Tomato Sauce, will be a repeat hit with friends and family.

1 Preheat the oven to 350°F and line two baking sheets with silicone baking mats or parchment paper. Cut off the tops and bottoms of the eggplants and peel. Trim the sides to create uniform rectangles. Using a knife (or mandoline), cut lengthwise to create ¼-inch slices. Spread the slices on the prepared baking sheets (it's okay if they overlap a little) and bake for 15 minutes until the eggplant is soft and pliable.

2 Meanwhile, in a large bowl, combine the chopped kale and the Tofu Ricotta. Mix with your hands until evenly combined. Set aside.

3 Spread a thin layer of tomato sauce on the bottoms of two glass or ceramic baking dishes, one 9 × 13-inch dish and one 9 × 9-inch dish. Add just enough sauce to coat the bottom, as though you are spreading sauce on a pizza.

4 Place an eggplant slice on a work surface. Place a heaping tablespoon of the ricotta mixture at one end of the eggplant slice and roll it up tightly. Place the roll in the pan and continue until the eggplant slices are used up, keeping the rolls packed closely together. (You'll have enough ricotta to fill the large dish and part of the smaller dish.) Top the rolls with another layer of tomato sauce and sprinkle any leftover ricotta on top. Don't use too much sauce during baking; more can be added when serving, and too much will make the entire dish soggy.

5 Cover both dishes with foil and bake for 30 minutes; then remove the foil and bake for 20 minutes more. As the moisture evaporates, the flavors concentrate.

6 To serve, drizzle generously with extra sauce, and garnish with fresh basil, red pepper flakes, and Cashew Parmesan Sprinkle. Enjoy immediately.

✎ NOTES: Jarred pasta sauce can be substituted for a last-minute option, but it typically needs to be heated in a pan to reduce and thicken. You can get by with one 24-ounce jar of marinara sauce, but have two just in case. Our Grandma Marie's Tomato Sauce makes this recipe special, so avoid store-bought sauce if possible.

For a bit of added decadence or an R&A, enjoy a sprinkle of vegan shredded parmesan cheese on top.

BAKED FALAFEL
with Lemon-Garlic Tahini Sauce

PREP TIME: **15 MINUTES**
PLUS OVERNIGHT SOAK
COOK TIME: **25 MINUTES**
YIELD: **6–8 SERVINGS**

INGREDIENTS

1 cup dry chickpeas, soaked in water overnight and rinsed

1 medium red onion, roughly chopped

2 tbsp fresh lemon juice

2 tbsp low-sodium tamari

3 garlic cloves, sliced

2 tsp ground cumin

1 tsp crushed red pepper flakes

1 cup fresh flat-leaf (Italian) parsley, stems removed

Pita bread (optional), to serve

For the sauce

4 tbsp tahini

2 tbsp freshly squeezed lemon juice

1 tsp minced garlic

¼ tsp smoked paprika

1 tsp minced fresh flat-leaf (Italian) parsley

This recipe delivers all the flavors of the favorite Middle Eastern staple, without the deep frying. Enjoy these enlightened patties in the traditional style—stuffed in a pita or wrapped in lavash with cucumbers, tomatoes, pickled vegetables, and tahini—or try them in our Falafel Salad (page 135).

1. Preheat the oven to 400°F. Line a baking sheet with parchment paper or a silicone baking mat and set aside.

2. In a food processor, combine the chickpeas and onions and process until smooth, stopping to scrape down the sides of the bowl as needed. Add the lemon juice, tamari, garlic, cumin, and red pepper flakes. Process until smooth. Pulse in the parsley until well distributed but still visible.

3. Using a cookie scoop, scoop the falafel mixture into small balls onto the prepared baking sheet. Place in the oven and bake for 20 to 25 minutes, until dark brown on the edges.

4. While the falafel is in the oven, combine all the sauce ingredients, except the parsley, in a small bowl. Stir until well combined, adding 4 to 6 tablespoons water as needed to achieve your desired thickness. Add the parsley and stir to combine.

5. Remove the falafel from the oven and serve with the tahini sauce inside a warm pita bread, on the Falafel Salad, or on their own. Leftover falafel can be refrigerated in an airtight container for up to 4 days.

✎ **NOTES:** Do not substitute canned chickpeas for the soaked dry chickpeas in this recipe; they will not yield the same texture.

To thin the sauce, add warm water 1 teaspoon at a time, stir, and adjust accordingly. Too much water may dilute the flavors, so if you make it thinner, you may need to add more lemon juice, garlic, smoked paprika, and parsley.

MEDITERRANEAN STUFFED PEPPERS
with Basil-Pine Nut Sauce

PREP TIME: **15 MINUTES**
  PLUS 30 MINUTES TO CHILL
COOK TIME: **60 MINUTES**
YIELD: **4–6 SERVINGS**

INGREDIENTS

6 bell peppers, any color

1lb asparagus, trimmed and cut into
  1-in pieces

2 cups cooked farro or brown rice

½ cup sun-dried tomatoes (not
  packed in oil), minced

3 tbsp tomato paste

1 cup minced red onion

2 tbsp minced black olives

2 tbsp basil chiffonade

1 tbsp pine nuts

1 tbsp capers

1 tbsp freshly squeezed lemon juice

2 tsp dried Italian seasoning blend

For the sauce

½ cup pine nuts

½ cup fresh basil, packed

¼ cup freshly squeezed lemon juice

1 tsp maple syrup

Nature's perfect edible cups filled with surprisingly savory, earthy, and hearty goodness. Farro is a nutty, chewy ancient grain that offers a unique twist to more commonly used whole grains. Sun-dried tomatoes and tomato paste add an umami undertone, olives and capers punch it up with brine, while pine nuts, lemon, and basil balance out the Mediterranean palate in this colorful recipe.

1   Preheat the oven to 400°F. Cut the peppers in half vertically (stem to base) and remove the seeds. Arrange the peppers cut-side-up in two 9 × 13-inch glass or ceramic baking dishes. Bake for 15 minutes and remove from the oven.

2   In a large bowl, combine the asparagus, cooked farro, sun-dried tomatoes, tomato paste, onions, olives, basil, pine nuts, capers, lemon juice, and Italian seasoning. Toss to combine. Spoon the farro mixture evenly into each pepper half. Cover with aluminum foil and bake for 40 to 45 minutes.

3   While the stuffed peppers are in the oven, prepare the sauce. In a blender, pulse the pine nuts until ground. Add the basil, lemon juice, and maple syrup, and blend. When the peppers are done, plate with a dollop of sauce and serve hot.

✎ **NOTE:** As an alternative to the pine nut and basil sauce, try Grandma Marie's Tomato Sauce (page 241).

BEAN BURGER FORMULATOR

PREP TIME: **20 MINUTES**
COOK TIME: **30 MINUTES**
YIELD: **6 PATTIES**

This flexible template for plant-based burgers starts with a simple bean and rice mixture. The flavor variations add fats, spices, and herbs that can be interchanged for your own creations.

INGREDIENTS

For the main burger mix:

1 (15oz) can beans of choice, drained and rinsed

1 cup cooked rice of choice

½ cup old-fashioned rolled oats

2 tbsp julienned sun-dried tomatoes (not packed in oil)

2 tsp ground flaxseed

½ tsp onion powder

½ tsp garlic powder

1 In a food processor, combine all the main burger ingredients, along with the ingredients for your burger flavor of choice (Hippie, Curry, Tex-Mex, BBQ, or Thai). Pulse a few times to distribute them through the bowl. Process for about 30 seconds until the mixture begins to form a ball. Stop and scrape the walls of the food processor. Mix again for 15 to 20 seconds.

2 Carefully remove the blade. (There shouldn't be much mix on it.) Use a spatula to gather the mixture together and transfer it to a bowl. Using your hands, gently compress the mixture into a ball. Place it back in the bowl, cover, and refrigerate for 30 minutes.

3 Preheat the oven to 375°F. Line a baking sheet with parchment paper. Form the mixture into 6 patties and place them on the prepared baking sheet. Bake for 30 minutes.

HIPPIE BURGER

(chickpeas/brown rice)

¼ cup hempseeds

2 tbsp nutritional yeast

2 tbsp **Magic Mushroom Powder** (page 242)

2 tbsp low-sodium tamari

2 tsp freshly squeezed lemon juice

2 cups finely chopped kale

Toppings: sliced avocado, sprouts, pickles, ketchup

CURRY BURGER

(chickpeas/brown rice)

2 tsp sweet curry powder

2 tbsp tomato paste

¼ cup loosely packed cilantro

¼ tsp garlic powder

1 tsp freshly squeezed lemon juice

1 tbsp low-sodium tahini

Toppings: cucumber raita or mango chutney

BBQ BURGER
(black beans/black rice)

1 tbsp chopped Medjool date

1 tsp molasses

¼ cup tomato paste

½ tsp smoked paprika

½ tsp cayenne

¼ tsp garlic powder

¼ tsp onion powder

1 tsp anchovy-free Worcestershire sauce

2 tsp apple cider vinegar

Toppings: **Coleslaw** (page 145), sautéed mushrooms and onions

THAI BURGER
(black beans/black rice)

¼ cup peanut butter

4 tsp freshly squeezed lime juice

1 tbsp Sriracha

1 tbsp low-sodium tamari

4 tsp **Magic Mushroom Powder** (page 242)

2 tbsp tamarind concentrate

Toppings: Sriracha, pickled vegetables

TEX-MEX BURGER
(black beans/black rice)

2 tsp chili powder

½ tsp smoked paprika

1 tbsp freshly squeezed lime juice

¼ cup diced red onion

¼ cup loosely packed cilantro

2 tbsp chopped jalapeño

Toppings: sliced avocado or guacamole, salsa

GARLIC MASHED POTATOES
with Magic Mushroom Gravy

PREP TIME: **15 MINUTES**
COOK TIME: **25 MINUTES**
YIELD: **4–8 SERVINGS**

INGREDIENTS

5lb Yukon Gold potatoes, chopped into uniform pieces (about 8 cups)

2 rosemary sprigs

2 thyme sprigs

1 bay leaf

1 cup diced yellow onion

4 garlic cloves, minced

1 cup unsweetened nondairy milk

1 tbsp low-sodium tamari

1 tsp freshly ground black pepper

For the gravy

1 cup diced yellow onion

8oz gourmet mushroom blend, sliced

1½ cups **Simple Stock** (page 96) or low-sodium vegetable broth

2 tbsp nutritional yeast

1 tbsp **Magic Mushroom Powder** (page 242)

2 tsp low-sodium tamari

1 tsp anchovy-free Worcestershire sauce

½ cup unsweetened nondairy milk

¼ tsp garlic powder

1 tbsp fresh rosemary, de-stemmed and chopped

1 tbsp fresh thyme, de-stemmed and chopped

½ tsp dry rubbed sage

2 tbsp cornstarch

½ tsp freshly squeezed lemon juice

Enjoy the goodness of Thanksgiving year-round, as these are easily sourced ingredients any time. We make enormous quantities of this recipe because we unabashedly love to tuck into hearty bowls of this classic comfort food. You can halve it if you must, but beware that you may wish you hadn't once you taste that first spoonful.

1 Place the potatoes in a 6-quart pot and fill with water until the potatoes are covered. Add the rosemary, thyme, and bay leaf. Bring to a boil over medium-high heat; then reduce heat and simmer for 15 to 20 minutes until fork-tender. Drain the water from the potatoes, and discard the rosemary and thyme stems and bay leaf. Set aside.

2 While the potatoes are cooking, prepare the gravy. Heat a large saucepan or Dutch oven over medium-high heat. Once hot, dry sauté the onions until they begin to brown, approximately 2 to 3 minutes. Add 1 tablespoon water and the mushrooms. Cover and cook the mushrooms until they release their liquid, about 2 minutes.

3 In a medium bowl, whisk together the vegetable broth, nutritional yeast, Magic Mushroom Powder, tamari, Worcestershire sauce, nondairy milk, and garlic powder. Add the mixture to the saucepan along with the rosemary, thyme, and rubbed sage. Reduce the heat and simmer for 2 to 3 minutes.

4 In a small bowl, whisk together the cornstarch and 1 tablespoon cold water to create a slurry. Add to the saucepan and stir gently for 2 to 3 minutes until the gravy thickens. Add the lemon juice and stir to combine. Remove from the heat, and set aside.

5 To complete the potatoes, heat another large saucepan or Dutch oven over medium-high heat. Once hot, dry sauté the onions until they begin to brown and turn translucent. If sautéing the garlic (see note), add to the pan with 1 tablespoon water and cook an additional 1 to 2 minutes, but don't burn the garlic. Remove from the heat.

6 In a large bowl, add the potatoes and begin to mash with a hand potato masher. When most of the pieces are smashed, add the nondairy milk and continue to mash and blend. (An immersion blender works well, too.) Once it begins to become smooth, mix in the onions, garlic, and tamari, and season with black pepper.

7 For each serving, scoop a huge spoonful of potatoes into a bowl and top with the gravy. Enjoy immediately.

✎ **NOTES:** For larger potatoes, quarter them lengthwise and then cut into 3 to 4 sections so they make equal-sized pieces that are ideal for mashing.

You can add more or less garlic, depending on your affinity for garlic. If you prefer raw garlic, you can add the cloves directly into the potatoes instead of sautéing them with the onions.

SHEPHERDESS PIE

PREP TIME: **20 MINUTES**
COOK TIME: **50 MINUTES**
YIELD: **4–6 SERVINGS**

INGREDIENTS

For the potato topping

2lb Yukon Gold potatoes, chopped into uniform pieces (about 4 cups)

2 rosemary sprigs

2 thyme sprigs

1 bay leaf

¼ cup unsweetened nondairy milk

1 tbsp nutritional yeast

¼ tsp garlic powder

⅛ tsp freshly ground black pepper

For the filling

2 cups diced red onion

½ cup finely diced celery

2 cups shredded carrots

1 cup minced shiitake mushrooms

3–5 garlic cloves, minced

½ cup low-sodium vegetable broth

¼ cup tomato paste

1 tbsp minced fresh rosemary

1 tbsp minced fresh thyme

1 cup cooked or canned black beans

1 cup cooked or canned lentils (green or brown)

1 cup frozen peas

2 tbsp low-sodium tamari

2 tbsp cornstarch

¼ cup red wine or vegetable broth

Traditionally, shepherd's pie consists of a savory meat filling covered with mashed potatoes. In this wholesome, meat-free "shepherdess" version, we combine lentils, beans, and meaty shiitakes with loads of veggies for a filling with huge savory flavor, and top it off with a blanket of creamy mashed potatoes.

1   Place the potatoes in a 6-quart pot and fill with water to an inch above the potatoes. Add the rosemary, thyme, and bay leaf. Bring to a boil over medium-high heat. Once boiling, reduce heat and simmer for 15 to 20 minutes, until the potatoes can be easily pierced with a fork.

2   Drain, reserving ¼ cup cooking water to start the mashing process. Discard the herb stems and bay leaf. In a large bowl, mash the potatoes using a potato masher or immersion blender with the reserved cooking water, nondairy milk, nutritional yeast, garlic powder, and pepper until smooth. Set aside.

3   Prepare the filling. Preheat the oven to 425°F. Heat a large saucepan or Dutch oven over medium-high heat. Once hot, sauté the onions, celery, and carrots with 1 to 2 tablespoons water for 3 to 4 minutes or until they begin to soften. Add the mushrooms and stir. Add the garlic and vegetable broth, stir, and let simmer for 60 to 90 seconds. Stir in the tomato paste, rosemary, thyme, black beans, lentils, and peas. Add the tamari and stir.

4   In a small bowl, whisk the cornstarch and wine to create a slurry. Add the slurry to the pan and continue cooking for 1 to 2 minutes or until the mixture has thickened and no liquid remains. Remove from heat.

5   Spoon the filling mixture into a 9 × 9-inch baking dish. Top with the mashed potatoes, using wet fingers to gently and evenly press over the filling. Once smooth, use your fingers to create an uneven surface (ripples and ridges) for optimal browning. Bake uncovered for 20 to 25 minutes, until the potatoes are golden brown. Serve hot over a bed of greens or enjoy on its own.

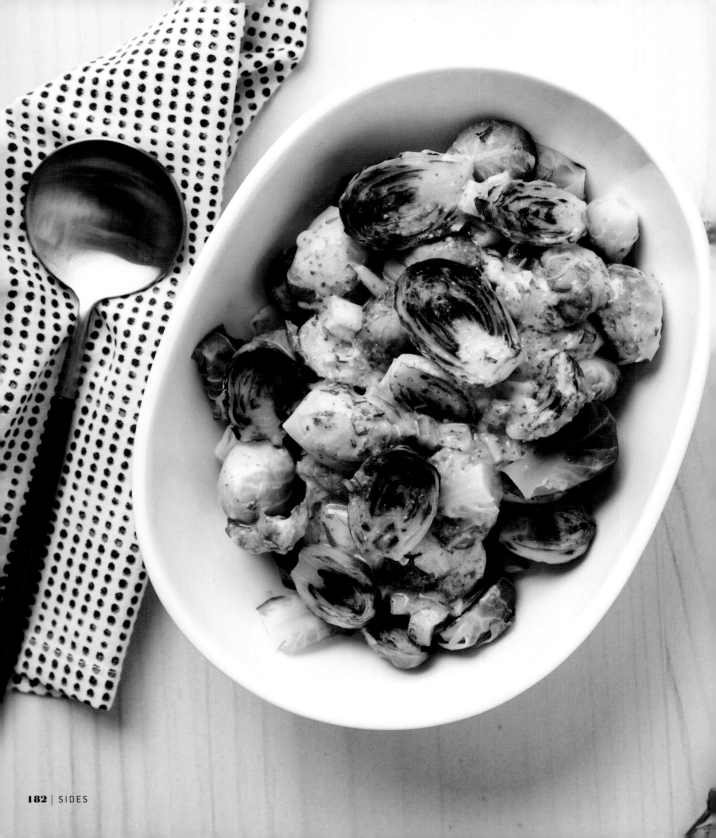

TARRAGON MUSTARD BRUSSELS SPROUTS

PREP TIME: **10 MINUTES**
COOK TIME: **15 MINUTES**
YIELD: **2 SERVINGS**

A tangy, fresh, and simple way to prepare Brussels sprouts. Resembling anise, tarragon offers a unique and bold taste that is enhanced by the acid and mustard in the sauce.

INGREDIENTS

1lb Brussels sprouts, ends trimmed

2 tbsp sliced shallot (about 1 medium shallot)

2 tbsp champagne or white wine vinegar

¼ cup coarse-ground mustard

1 tbsp roughly chopped fresh tarragon

Splash of freshly squeezed lemon juice

1   In a large stockpot, bring 4 cups water to a boil over high heat. Once boiling, carefully add the trimmed Brussels sprouts to the water and blanch for 3 to 4 minutes.

2   Meanwhile, in a small blender, combine the shallot, vinegar, mustard, and tarragon and pulse a couple of times, until well combined but not liquified. Set aside.

3   Drain the Brussels sprouts in a colander. Once cool enough to handle, slice into halves.

4   Heat a large sauté pan over high heat and place the Brussels sprouts in the pan, cut side down. Dry sauté the Brussels sprouts until they begin to brown, but don't overcook—they should stay crisp. Add water if needed to avoid burning.

5   Transfer Brussels sprouts to a large bowl and pour the sauce over top. Toss to combine. Drizzle lemon juice on top, or plate with a lemon wedge, and serve hot.

CAULIFLOWER RICE CHICKPEA CURRY

PREP TIME: **20 MINUTES**
COOK TIME: **15 MINUTES**
YIELD: **2 SERVINGS**

INGREDIENTS

4 cups cauliflower florets (from 1 medium head cauliflower)

1 cup diced onion

3 garlic cloves, sliced thick

1 (28oz) can petite diced tomatoes

1 (15oz) can chickpeas, drained and rinsed

1 tbsp curry powder

1 cup chopped kale

1 cup (loosely packed) fresh cilantro, de-stemmed and roughly chopped

¼–½ tsp cayenne, to taste

1 tbsp freshly squeezed lemon juice

1 tbsp low-sodium tamari

One creative and adaptable way to add more cruciferous vegetables to your meals and save time in the kitchen is to replace rice in a recipe with riced cauliflower. You can use a food processor (as we do here), a box grater, or a potato ricer, or simply purchase the convenient bags of pre-riced cauliflower in the refrigerated or freezer sections at the store. This is a satisfying, colorful curry dish full of zing and zest that is quick and easy to prepare.

1 In a food processor, pulse the cauliflower florets into rice. (This may need to be done in batches, depending on the size of your food processer bowl.)

2 Heat a large saucepan or Dutch oven over medium-high heat. Once hot, sauté the onions with as little water as possible—just enough to avoid burning—until they begin to brown, 3 to 4 minutes. Add the garlic and sauté for 30 to 60 seconds, or until the garlic is lightly browned, being careful not to scorch.

3 Add the cauliflower rice, tomatoes, chickpeas, and curry powder, and stir to combine. Cover and simmer for 3 to 4 minutes. Add the kale, cover, and simmer for 3 to 4 minutes more. Add the cilantro, cayenne pepper, lemon juice, and tamari, and toss to combine. Enjoy immediately.

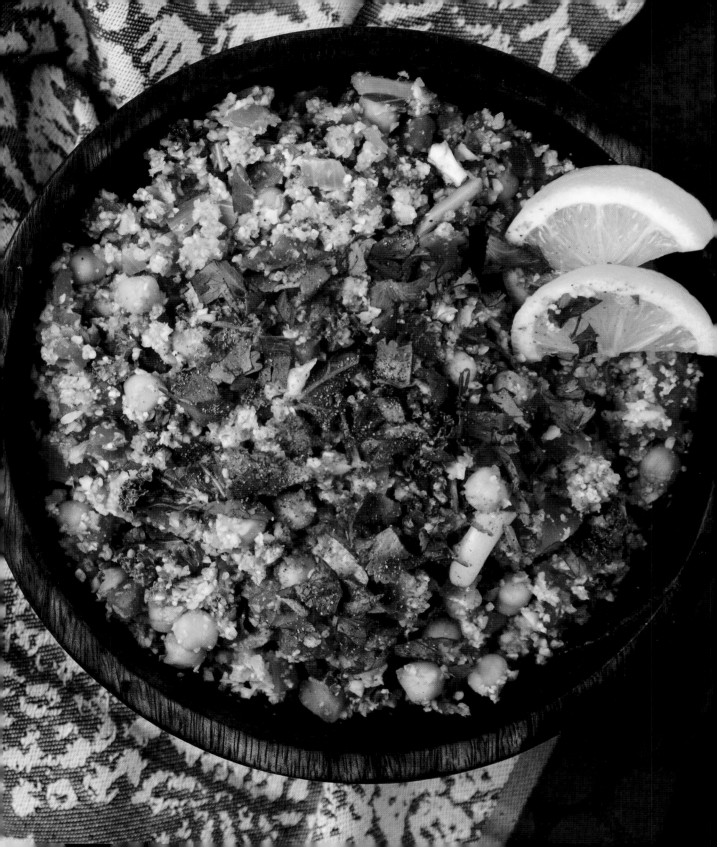

NEW YEAR'S COLLARD GREENS

PREP TIME: **15 MINUTES**
COOK TIME: **15 MINUTES**
YIELD: **4 SERVINGS**

INGREDIENTS

4 bunches collard greens

2 medium yellow onions, sliced thick into half-circles

¼ cup apple cider vinegar, divided

1–2 tsp molasses, to taste

Hot sauce (optional), to taste

Celebrating New Year's in the South is the perfect excuse to eat more greens. Because collards are green, they symbolize money, and are enjoyed along with black-eyed peas for financial prosperity in the New Year. Of course, this tasty traditional dish can be enjoyed anywhere in the world and on any day of the year.

1 Wash the collard greens well. Stack 5 or 6 leaves at a time and roll tightly from the long side to create a long, cigar-like cylinder. Slice crosswise into ¼-inch-thick ribbons. Set aside.

2 Heat a large saucepan over medium-high heat. Sauté the onions with ¼ cup water until brown, approximately 5 to 10 minutes. Add 2 tablespoons apple cider vinegar and 1 tsp molasses and stir to combine.

3 Add the collard greens to the pan along with the remaining 2 tablespoons apple cider vinegar. Toss well to combine. Cook, covered, for 5 minutes, until the greens are tender and not bitter.

4 Adjust the sweet and sour flavors with molasses and apple cider vinegar. It should have a hint of sour and not too much sweetness. Stir in a dash of hot sauce, if desired, and plate. Drizzle with hot sauce, as desired, to serve.

✎ **NOTE:** We like our collard greens al dente. If you prefer them more tender, add approximately 1 cup low-sodium vegetable broth to the pan and cook for up to 20 minutes, covered.

NEW YEAR'S BLACK-EYED PEAS

PREP TIME: **5 MINUTES
PLUS OVERNIGHT SOAK**
COOK TIME: **1 HOUR 30 MINUTES**
YEILD: **4 SERVINGS**

INGREDIENTS

1 cup diced yellow onion

½ cup thinly sliced celery

2 tbsp minced jalapeño

2 garlic cloves, minced

1 red bell pepper, chopped

8 cups **Simple Stock** (page 96) or
low-sodium vegetable broth

1 lb dried black-eyed peas, soaked
overnight and drained

3 bay leaves

1 tbsp chopped fresh thyme

Freshly ground black pepper,
to taste

¼–½ tsp liquid smoke, to taste

We love the Southern tradition of eating black-eyed peas—also known as "Hoppin' John"—on New Year's Day for prosperity in the upcoming year. Instead of pork, we infuse classic flavor into the expanding legumes (a symbol for expanding wealth) with plenty of spices and a dash or so of liquid smoke.

1 Heat a large saucepan or Dutch oven over medium-high heat. Once hot, sauté the onions and celery with as little water as possible—just enough to avoid burning—for about 5 minutes or until they begin to brown.

2 Add the jalapeño, garlic, and bell pepper, and sauté for 30 to 60 seconds or until the garlic is lightly browned, taking care not to scorch.

3 Add the broth, black-eyed peas, bay leaves, thyme, and black pepper. Bring to a boil. Lower the heat, partially cover, and simmer for 90 minutes, until the peas are soft. Add the liquid smoke and more pepper, if desired, to taste. Remove the bay leaves and serve warm over our New Year's Collard Greens (page 186).

SRIRACHA STUFFED MUSHROOMS

PREP TIME: **15 MINUTES**
COOK TIME: **40 MINUTES**
YIELD: **4 SERVINGS**

INGREDIENTS

24oz baby bella mushrooms

½ cup raw cashews

3 tbsp nutritional yeast

1 cup roughly chopped red bell pepper

2 garlic cloves, minced

3 tbsp Sriracha

2 tbsp freshly squeezed lemon juice

This was one of our very first recipe creations as a team, and it is now a party favorite. With Ray's nickname for Julieanna being "Nooch" due to her love of nutritional yeast, Sriracha as a choice condiment on almost everything, and mushrooms as one of our mutually favorite foods, these spicy, decadent bites of umami cover all the bases. Serve these to guests, or eat them all yourself. By using the mushroom stems in the stuffing, we've trimmed the waste to keep your waist trim.

1 Preheat the oven to 350°F and line a baking sheet with parchment paper.

2 Wipe the mushrooms with a moist paper towel or soft brush and remove the stems. Dice the stems and set aside in a medium bowl. Place the mushroom caps on the prepared baking sheet.

3 In a blender, pulse the cashews and nutritional yeast to a fine powder. (Do not over blend.) Scrape the corners of the blender with a spatula to make sure all the powder is free. Add the bell pepper, garlic, Sriracha, and lemon juice and blend until fully combined and creamy. If it is too thick, a small amount of water can be added, but take care not make it too thin and runny.

4 Add the sauce to the bowl with the mushroom stems and gently stir to combine. Spoon the mixture evenly into each mushroom cap.

5 Bake in the oven for 25 to 30 minutes or until the filling is firm and golden and the mushrooms have released most of their liquid. Serve hot.

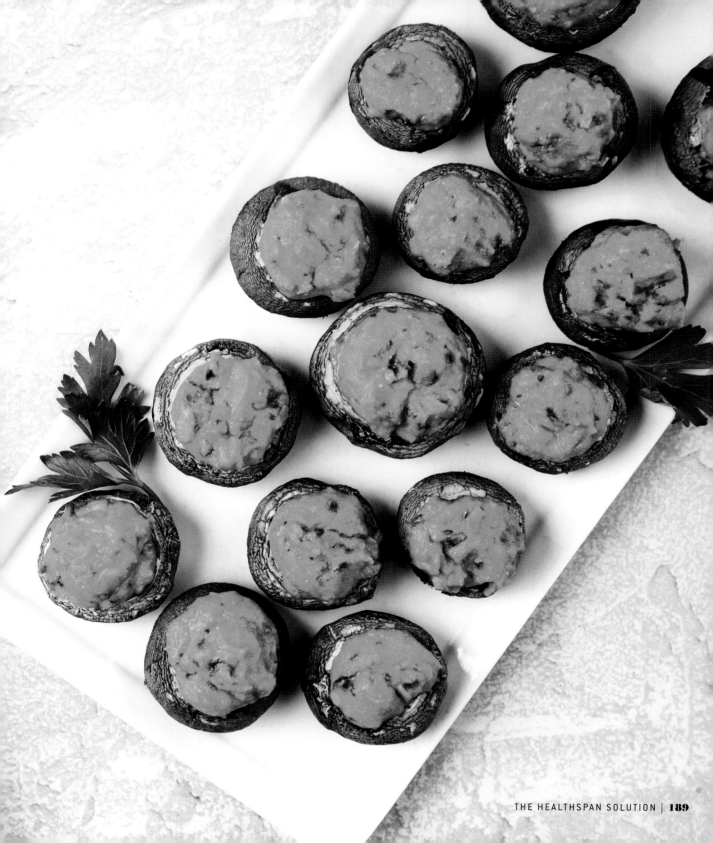

TROPICAL BLACK BEANS AND CORN
with Chili-Lime Dressing

PREP TIME: **30 MINUTES**
COOK TIME: **5 MINUTES**
YIELD: **2 SERVINGS**

INGREDIENTS

1 cup corn kernels, fresh or frozen

1 (15oz) can black beans, drained and rinsed

2 cups chopped mango

1¾ cups chopped papaya

1 cup diced red bell pepper

1 cup halved cherry tomatoes

½ cup chopped fresh cilantro

¼ cup minced red onion

2 tbsp minced jalapeño

For the dressing

3–4 green olives

¼ cup chopped papaya

2 tbsp freshly squeezed lime juice

2 tsp chili powder

This colorful dish features velvety black beans, sweet roasted corn, mango, papaya, sweet red peppers, cherry tomatoes, and just a hint of jalapeño heat. Try it as a filling for a corn tortilla wrap or toss it on top of some greens for a deliciously satisfying meal. For the chili-lime dressing, we use a few green olives and papaya instead of the olive oil and sugar found in many recipes. It's delicious served both warm or chilled.

1 Heat a large saucepan over medium-high heat. Once hot, add the corn and toast for about 5 minutes, until the kernels start to pop and are browned, stirring occasionally.

2 To make the dressing, combine all ingredients in a blender and process until smooth.

3 In a large serving bowl, combine the roasted corn, black beans, mango, papaya, bell pepper, cherry tomatoes, cilantro, red onion, and jalapeños. Pour the dressing over and toss to combine. Garnish with additional cilantro, if desired, and enjoy immediately.

✎ **NOTE:** To save time, you can substitute frozen mango and papaya chunks for fresh. Thaw and drain excess liquid before using.

MEXICAN RICE

PREP TIME: **5 MINUTES**
COOK TIME: **40 MINUTES**
YIELD: **4 SERVINGS**

INGREDIENTS

2 cups **Simple Stock** (page 96) or
   low-sodium vegetable broth

¼ cup tomato paste

1 cup uncooked long-grain
   brown rice

1 cup finely diced yellow onion

1 medium jalapeño, de-seeded and
   diced

½ tsp dried Mexican oregano

¾ tsp ground cumin

¾ tsp chili powder

Fresh cilantro, chopped, to serve

Freshly squeezed lime juice,
   to serve

Simply lovely side dish served al dente with Mexican-inspired spiced tomato flavors. Enjoy on its own or as the base for the Mexican Rice Burrito Bowl (page 155).

1 In a quart-sized measuring cup or medium bowl, whisk together the vegetable broth and tomato paste.

2 Heat a large saucepan over medium-high heat. Once hot, add the rice and toast for 2 to 3 minutes, until the grains start to pop, stirring constantly. Add the onions and jalapeño and continue to stir. Cook for 3 to 5 minutes or until they begin to brown.

3 Stir in the oregano, cumin, and chili powder. Add the vegetable broth and tomato paste mixture and bring to a boil over high heat. Once boiling, reduce heat to low, cover, and simmer for 30 minutes until all the liquid has been absorbed. Stir, remove from heat, and let sit covered for 5 to 10 minutes.

4 Before serving, add the cilantro and lime juice to taste and enjoy immediately.

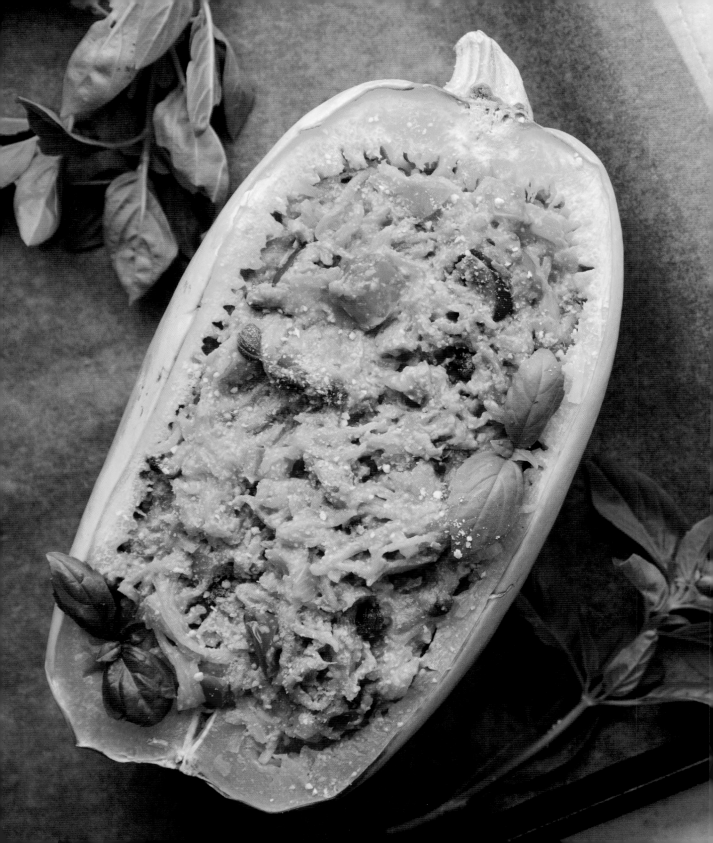

SPAGHETTI SQUASH PUTTANESCA

PREP TIME: **15 MINUTES**
COOK TIME: **90 MINUTES**
YIELD: **2 SERVINGS**

INGREDIENTS

1 medium-sized spaghetti squash, cut in half and de-seeded

¼ cup raw cashews

2 tbsp nutritional yeast

¼ cup unsweetened nondairy milk

½ cup diced yellow onion

2 garlic cloves, minced

½ cup chopped tomatoes

¼ cup tomato paste

1 tbsp Kalamata olives, pitted and chopped

1 tbsp capers

¼–½ tsp crushed red pepper flakes, to taste

1 tbsp basil chiffonade, to garnish

Cashew Parmesan Sprinkle (optional, page 239), to garnish

Apparently, the etymology of puttanesca can be translated from Italian to mean either "prostitutes" or "anchovies, olives, and capers" in English. Whether or not it's accurate that this robust tomato sauce originated as a dish to lure clients in off the streets with its aroma, its classic combination of ingredients and straightforward preparation is worthwhile. Swapping spaghetti squash for pasta minimizes the energy density while enhancing the nutrition, fun, and flavor as it is the perfect delivery system for this sassy sauce.

1   Preheat the oven to 350°F. Line a baking sheet with parchment paper or a silicone baking mat. Place both halves of the spaghetti squash on the prepared baking sheet, cut side down. Bake for 40 to 60 minutes or until the flesh is tender and the edges are golden brown. Remove from the oven to cool. Once cool enough to handle, scrape out the flesh with a fork to create spaghetti-like strands, reserving the shells to serve. Set aside.

2   In a blender, pulse the cashews and nutritional yeast until a fine powder forms, 10 to 20 seconds. Add the nondairy milk and blend until smooth, 30 to 60 seconds. Set aside.

3   Heat a medium saucepan over medium-high heat. Sauté the onions with 1 to 2 tablespoons water until they are translucent. Add the garlic and sauté for 30 to 60 seconds or until golden, taking care not to scorch.

4   Add the tomatoes, tomato paste, and ¼ cup water, and stir. Add the olives, capers, and red pepper flakes, and heat for 1 minute more. Toss in the spaghetti squash strands and cashew cream, stir to combine, and remove from the heat.

5   To serve, scoop the mixture into the reserved squash shells. Garnish with basil and Cashew Parmesan Sprinkle, if using, and enjoy immediately.

BAKED SWEET POTATOES
with Pistachio Gremolata

PREP TIME: **10 MINUTES**
COOK TIME: **40–60 MINUTES**
YIELD: **2 POTATOES**

INGREDIENTS

2 medium sweet potatoes

½ cup chopped raw pistachios

2 tbsp finely chopped flat-leaf (Italian) parsley

2 tbsp finely chopped fresh cilantro

2 tbsp finely chopped fresh mint leaves

1 tbsp orange zest

1 tbsp lemon zest

1 tbsp freshly squeezed orange juice

1 tsp freshly squeezed lemon juice

2–3 green olives, minced

1 garlic clove, minced

⅛–¼ tsp crushed red pepper flakes (optional)

Italian in origin, gremolata is a pesto-like condiment made with fresh herbs, citrus zest, and garlic. In this recipe, we punch up the flavor with olives and a dash of heat from red pepper flakes and serve it over a perfectly baked sweet potato. This is surprisingly filling for those days when you need a little extra comfort and elegance all in one.

1. Preheat the oven to 400°F. Line a baking sheet with a silicone baking mat or parchment paper. Scrub the potatoes and poke a few holes in the flesh with a fork. Place on the prepared baking sheet and bake for 40 to 60 minutes, until juices begin to seep out and they are easily pierced with a toothpick or knife.

2. While the potatoes are in the oven, heat a medium saucepan over medium-high heat. Once hot, add the pistachios and toast for 3 to 5 minutes, until fragrant.

3. In a medium bowl, combine the toasted pistachios, parsley, cilantro, mint, orange zest, lemon zest, orange juice, lemon juice, olives, garlic, and red pepper flakes, if using. Mix well. Serve over the baked sweet potatoes.

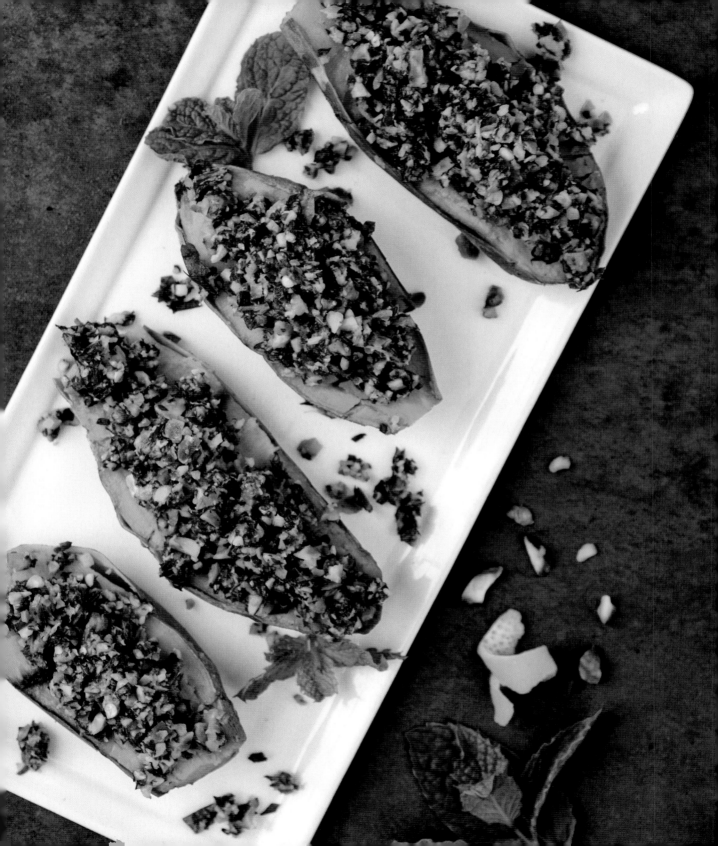

SIZZLING BALSAMIC ROASTED VEGETABLES

PREP TIME: **15 MINUTES**
COOK TIME: **30 MINUTES**
YIELD: **2 SERVINGS**

INGREDIENTS

1 small head cauliflower, cut into florets (see note)

1½ cups halved Brussels sprouts

1 cup peeled and halved shallots (if large, cut into quarters)

1 cup sliced parsnips

1 cup chopped red bell pepper

¼ cup balsamic vinegar

1 tsp Dijon mustard

1 tbsp minced fresh thyme

There's plenty of sizzle and sass in this colorful collection of cruciferous vegetables! Although it may seem like a whole lot of vegetables when they first go in the oven, they shrink as they caramelize while roasting, making them irresistible and quick to consume. Dressed simply over some salad greens, this a meal that explodes with both nutrition and flavor.

1 Preheat the oven to 425°F and line a baking sheet with a silicone baking mat or parchment paper. Place a cast iron griddle or pan in the oven and allow it to heat while the vegetables roast.

2 Spread the cauliflower, Brussels sprouts, shallots, parsnips, and bell pepper on the prepared baking sheet. Place in the oven and roast for 30 minutes or until the vegetables begin to caramelize and brown at the edges.

3 While the vegetables roast, in a small saucepan over medium-low heat, combine the balsamic vinegar and mustard and bring to a simmer. Simmer for 3 to 5 minutes until the liquid has reduced to approximately half the volume, stirring frequently. Add the thyme and simmer for another 1 to 2 minutes. Remove from heat.

4 Remove the skillet from the oven and place on a potholder. Scoop all the vegetables into the skillet and toss with the balsamic reduction. Serve hot and sizzling as a side or over salad greens, tossed with an extra splash of balsamic.

NOTE: You can use any color cauliflower or a blend of different colors, depending on what is available locally and seasonally. Try experimenting with colors like purple and yellow for a vibrantly hued dish.

SWISS CHARD AND MUSHROOMS

with Lemon-Tahini Date Sauce

PREP TIME: **15 MINUTES**
COOK TIME: **10 MINUTES**
YIELD: **2 SERVINGS**

INGREDIENTS

2 cups diced yellow onion

2 cups sliced shiitake
  mushroom caps

4 cups chopped Swiss chard,
  stems removed

1 garlic clove

3 tbsp freshly squeezed lemon juice

2 Medjool dates, pitted (see note)

2 tbsp pine nuts, divided

1 tbsp tahini

½ tsp za'atar

1 cup cooked brown rice

Do you have greens growing in your garden? Or are they merely abundant in the store at the right season? Take advantage of the most health-promoting, nutrient-dense food groups (go greens!) with this edgy, seriously sour, simple stir-fry. Za'atar is a savory spice mixture traditionally used in the Middle East and, together with the tahini, lemon, and garlic, offers a deep, delicious, and complex flavor profile.

1 Heat a large saucepan or Dutch oven over medium-high heat. Once hot, dry sauté the onions until they begin to brown, about 2 minutes. Add the mushrooms on top of the onions, cover, and steam for an additional 2 to 3 minutes. Stir, then add the chard on top with 1 tablespoon water. Cover and steam for 3 to 4 minutes until the chard is tender but not soggy.

2 While the vegetables cook, in a blender, combine the garlic, lemon juice, dates, 1 tablespoon pine nuts, tahini, za'atar, and 1 tablespoon warm water. Blend until the dates and garlic are puréed.

3 Pack the rice into a measuring cup for a mold and plate in the center of a serving bowl. Surround the rice with the cooked chard, onions, and mushrooms. Drizzle the sauce over the greens and rice. Garnish with the remaining pine nuts and serve immediately.

✎ **NOTE:** This is tart, but you can amp up the sweetness with more dates if desired. For extra flavor, toast the pine nuts in a saucepan over medium-high heat for 1 to 2 minutes or until fragrant.

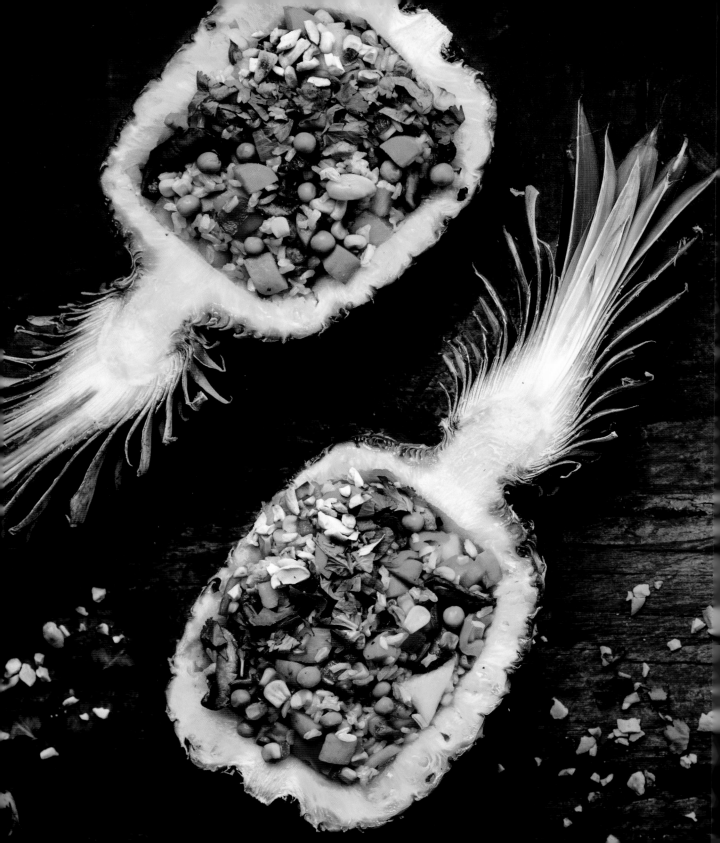

PINEAPPLE FRIED RICE

PREP TIME: **35 MINUTES**
COOK TIME: **15 MINUTES**
YIELD: **2–4 SERVINGS**

INGREDIENTS

1 medium pineapple

1 cup corn kernels

½ cup diced red onion

4oz gourmet mushroom blend, sliced

1 cup diced carrots

1 cup peas

1 cup diced red bell pepper

2 tsp low-sodium tamari

2 cups cooked brown rice

1 tbsp freshly squeezed lime juice

2 tbsp crushed raw cashews

½ cup minced fresh cilantro

1 tsp Sriracha

Thailand is known as "the land of smiles," and in our many trips there teaching plant-based culinary retreats, we never miss a chance to order pineapple fried rice. Don't worry, once you've scooped out a couple of pineapples, it's not that difficult. (And though these are extra fancy, you don't have to use the shells as serving dishes; you really just need its fruit.) Pick a pineapple with just a little give and a fragrant pineapple smell at the bottom. After your first bite, you'll surely feel that Thailand smile take hold.

1 Preheat the oven to 350°F. Line a baking sheet with a silicone baking mat or parchment paper.

2 Using a large, sharp knife, cut the pineapple lengthwise through the leaves into two halves. Remove the flesh from each half to create pineapple "bowls." Use a serrated knife to cut around the perimeter of each pineapple half, leaving about ¼ inch at the edge. Cut out the center core of the pineapple, and then use a spoon to scoop the flesh and juice into a medium bowl. Chop the flesh into ½-inch pieces. Reserve 1½ cups chopped pineapple for the filling and set aside. (Any remaining pineapple can be reserved for another use.)

3 Wrap the green pineapple leaves with aluminum foil to prevent burning and place the pineapple bowls on the prepared baking sheet, cut side up. Bake for 5 minutes, remove from the oven, and set aside. (Baking dries out the skin to make a firmer bowl.)

4 Heat a large wok or saucepan over medium-high heat. Once hot, add the corn and roast for 2 to 3 minutes until it begins to brown, stirring occasionally. Add the onions and sauté for another minute. Add the mushrooms along with 1 tablespoon water. Cover and steam until the mushrooms release their liquid and soften, 2 to 3 minutes. Stir in the carrots, peas, and bell pepper and mix well. Cover and cook for another 3 to 4 minutes. Add the tamari, 1½ cups pineapple, rice, and lime juice, and toss to combine.

5 Meanwhile, toast the cashews in a hot, dry pan over medium-high heat until browned.

6 Remove the pineapple rice from the heat and stir in the cilantro and Sriracha. Spoon into the pineapple shells, mounding high, top with the toasted cashews, and enjoy immediately.

✎ **NOTE:** Of course, using the pineapple shell as a serving dish is optional, but it is nice if you are entertaining. For a quick shortcut, simply use 1½ cups pineapple chunks, either from a can, defrosted from frozen, or fresh.

VEGETABLE FRIED RICE

PREP TIME: **20 MINUTES**
COOK TIME: **15 MINUTES**
YIELD: **4 SERVINGS**

INGREDIENTS

2 cups diced yellow onion

2 cups thinly sliced shiitake mushroom caps

1 small zucchini, sliced thick and quartered

4 cups broccoli florets

1 cup chopped red bell pepper

2 tsp sesame oil

4 garlic cloves, minced

2 tbsp minced fresh ginger root

3 cups cooked brown rice

½ cup frozen shelled edamame, defrosted

2 cups chopped kale

2–3 tbsp low-sodium tamari

2 scallions, thinly sliced, to garnish

½–1 tsp nori flakes, to garnish

Enjoy all of the fried without all the grease. You may be surprised by how far a couple teaspoons of sesame oil can go toward total decadence. This dish is studded with a gorgeous array of vegetables and edamame and is a substantial, satisfying, and salubrious alternative to take out.

1   Heat a wok or large saucepan over medium-high heat. Once hot, dry sauté the onions until they begin to brown, 1 to 2 minutes. Add the mushrooms, cover, and cook for 1 minute more. Add the zucchini, broccoli, bell pepper, and 1 tablespoon water. Stir, cover, and cook for 2 to 4 minutes.

2   Push the vegetables to the edges of the wok, creating an opening in the center. Drop the sesame oil into that center, followed by the garlic and ginger. Heat for 30 to 60 seconds, until golden brown. Toss to combine all ingredients.

3   Add the cooked rice and edamame, and toss to combine. Place the kale on top along with 1 tablespoon water, cover, and cook for 2 minutes. Stir in the kale, scraping the bottom, cover, and continue steaming for 2 minutes more. Add the tamari and toss to combine. Remove from the heat.

4   To serve, garnish with the scallions and nori flakes. Enjoy immediately.

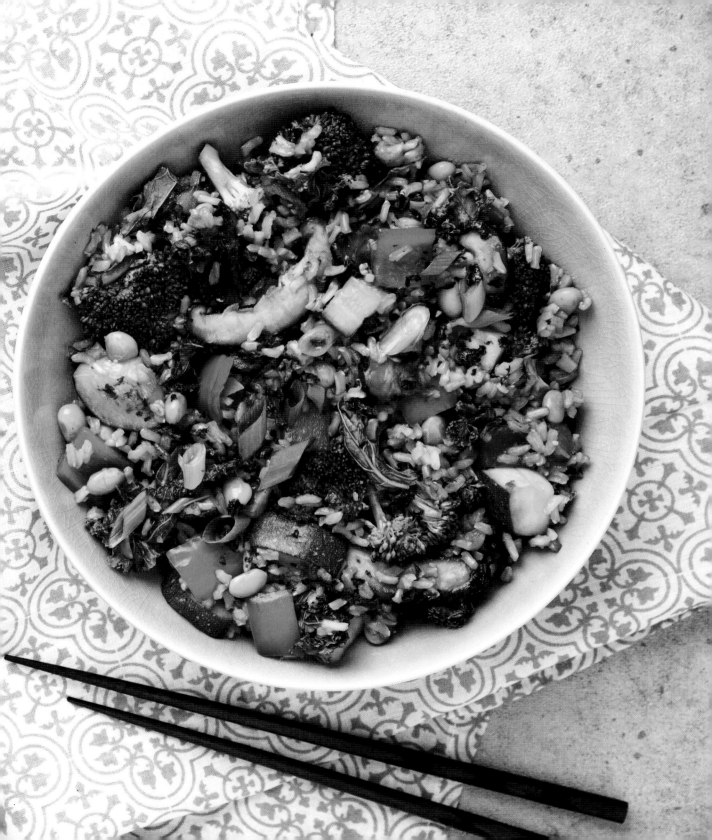

SPICY BLACK BEANS AND MANGOES

PREP TIME: **10 MINUTES**
COOK TIME: **10 MINUTES**
YIELD: **1–2 SERVINGS**

INGREDIENTS

1 cup diced red onion

1 (15oz) can black beans, drained and rinsed

1 cup chopped mango

2 tbsp thinly sliced jalapeño

½ tsp chipotle powder or ancho powder

¼ tsp ground cumin

¼ tsp dried Mexican oregano

¼ tsp freshly ground black pepper

1 tbsp freshly squeezed lime juice, plus more to taste

¼ cup chopped fresh cilantro (optional)

Quick, spicy, and deliciously sweet, this dish is a great last-minute, hearty meal. Keeping items such as canned beans and frozen mango stocked in the kitchen makes prep extra easy. Pro tip: Combining vitamin C-rich foods with iron-rich foods—as in the mango with black beans here—enhances absorption of the iron.

1   In a large saucepan over medium-high heat, dry sauté the onions with as little water as possible—just enough to avoid burning but still allow browning on the bottom of the pan—until the onions are translucent. Add the black beans, mango, jalapeño, chipotle, cumin, oregano, and black pepper. Cook over medium-high heat, stirring occasionally, for 5 to 10 minutes.

2   Remove from heat and add the fresh lime juice before serving. Sprinkle with the cilantro, if using. Serve warm in a bowl or over a bed of greens, a baked potato, rice, or quinoa.

MANGO ROASTED CORN SALSA

PREP TIME: **10 MINUTES**
COOK TIME: **6 MINUTES**
YIELD: **4 SERVINGS**

INGREDIENTS

1 cup corn kernels

2 cups diced mango

1 cup halved cherry tomatoes

¼ cup finely diced red onion

2 tbsp freshly squeezed lime juice

½ tsp chili powder

1 tbsp seasoned rice vinegar

¼ cup chopped fresh cilantro leaves

This salsa is a festive blend of sweet, sour, and spicy with a whole lot of "fresh." We created it to serve with the Fajita Salad (page 151), but decided it was too delicious to not be presented as a standalone treat or condiment for many other dishes. Take it to a tailgate party or serve it at a cookout on Cinco de Mayo with toasted tortillas.

1   Heat a saucepan over medium-high heat and add the corn. Dry roast the corn until golden brown, 3 to 6 minutes, stirring frequently to avoid burning.

2   In a serving bowl, toss the roasted corn with all remaining ingredients. Serve over rice, as a cabbage wrap, in the Fajita Salad (page 151), on a burrito, or on its own with a spoon.

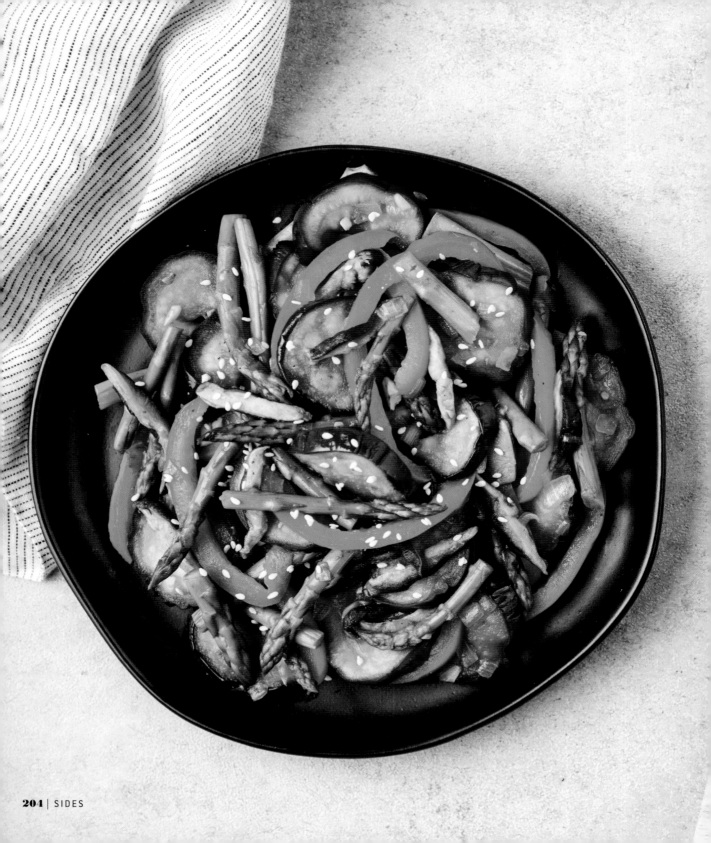

SPICY SESAME ASPARAGUS AUBERGINE

PREP TIME: **15 MINUTES**
COOK TIME: **15 MINUTES**
YIELD: **2 SERVINGS**

INGREDIENTS

1 cup diced sweet yellow onion

4 cups sliced Chinese eggplant

5oz shiitake mushroom caps, sliced

1lb trimmed asparagus, cut into
 2-in pieces

1 cup sliced red bell pepper

¼ cup raw cashews, crushed

1 tbsp toasted sesame oil

3 garlic cloves, minced

1 tbsp low-sodium tamari

1 tsp Sriracha

Aubergine—eggplant—is essentially "free food" as it is very high in fiber, low in energy, and versatile due to its spongy texture that sops up surrounding flavors. This recipe shows how to effectively use oil as an ingredient to optimize cooking and flavors without being burdensome, maximizing the pungent aroma that is the hallmark of toasted sesame oil.

1   Heat a wok or large saucepan over medium-high heat. When hot, add the onions and dry sauté until they begin to brown and are translucent, approximately 5 minutes. Add the eggplant, mushrooms, and 2 tablespoons water. Cover and let steam for 5 minutes.

2   Stir and add the asparagus, bell pepper, and another 2 tablespoons water. Cover again and steam for 4 to 5 more minutes, but avoid overcooking.

3   Meanwhile, heat a small saucepan over medium-high heat. Once hot, place the cashews in the pan and toast for 1 to 2 minutes until browned, stirring constantly to avoid scorching. Remove from heat and set aside.

4   When the asparagus is tender but still crisp, remove the lid. Push the vegetables to the edges of the wok, creating an opening in the center. Drop the sesame oil into that center, followed by the garlic. Heat for 30 to 60 seconds. Toss to combine all ingredients. Add the tamari and Sriracha, and stir once more. Garnish with the toasted cashews and enjoy immediately.

MANGO AVOCADO SPRING ROLLS

PREP TIME: **25 MINUTES**
COOK TIME: **NONE**
YIELD: **8 ROLLS**

INGREDIENTS

8 (8-inch) round rice paper
  wrappers

For the dressing

1 tsp minced fresh ginger

¼ cup chopped mango

½ medium orange, peeled and
  seeds removed

¼ cup loosely packed fresh cilantro

1 tbsp chopped fresh mint

1 tbsp minced shallots

2 tsp freshly squeezed lime juice

1 tsp low-sodium tamari

For the filling

1 cup shredded red cabbage

1 cup shredded romaine lettuce

1 cup thinly sliced avocado

1 cup julienned English (hothouse)
  cucumber

1 cup julienned jicama

1 cup julienned mango

¼ cup fresh cilantro leaves, whole
  cup fresh mint leaves, whole

Sriracha, optional

Fresh spring rolls are wonderful to eat and even more fun to make. Here, we've used cucumber, cabbage, jicama, romaine, and mango, but feel free to mix and match your favorite fresh veggies, herbs, and fruits. Our dipping sauce is pungent, citrusy, and fresh, with tropical flavors from mango, cilantro, and mint.

1   Make the dressing. In a blender, combine the ginger, mango, orange, cilantro, mint, shallots, lime juice, tamari, and 2 tablespoons water. Blend until smooth and set aside.

2   Gather all the filling ingredients on a large plate or in separate bowls. Fill a large, shallow bowl with warm water. Place 1 spring roll wrapper in the bowl for 3 to 4 seconds to soften. (The wrapper should still be firm when you start, because it softens further as water soaks in.)

3   Lay the wet wrapper flat on a large work surface. (Be prepared to work fast, as wrappers get soggy and sticky quickly.) In a row across the bottom third of the wrapper, place equal portions of the filling ingredients, leaving about 1 inch on each side. Drizzle a little dressing on top (and Sriracha, if using). Fold the bottom of the wrapper up over the filling and roll tightly until you reach the middle of the wrap. Fold the sides inward, place a few cilantro and mint leaves at the top of the wrapper, and continue to roll until you reach the top.

4   Repeat with the remaining ingredients. Serve immediately with the remaining dressing as a dipping sauce.

✎ **NOTE:** The key to spring roll success is good timing when hydrating the rice paper. If it becomes too wet, it sticks and rips, but if left too dry, it is brittle and breaks. Prepare your filling ingredients first and be sure to have them handy when the rice paper is ready.

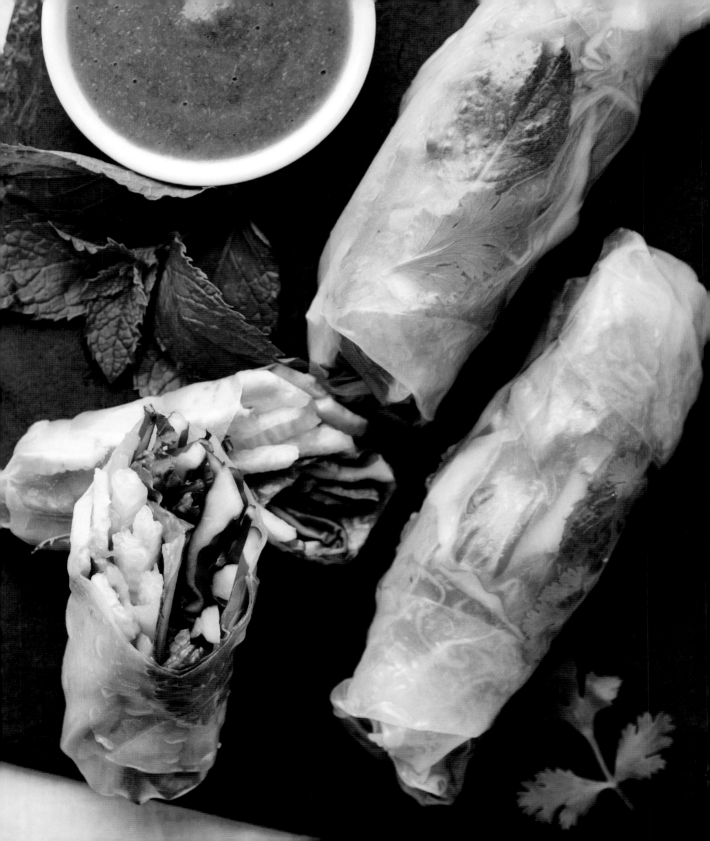

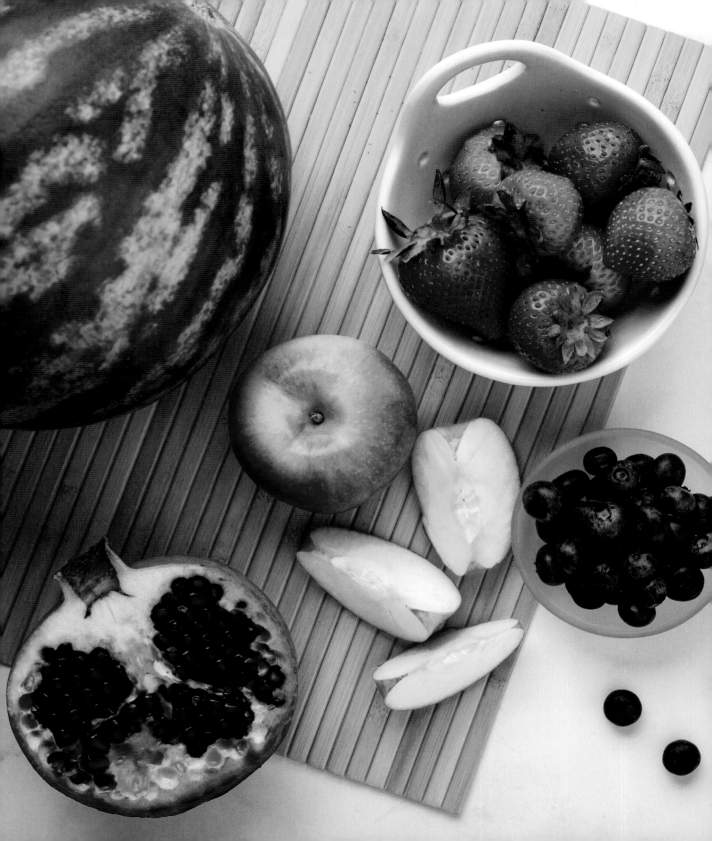

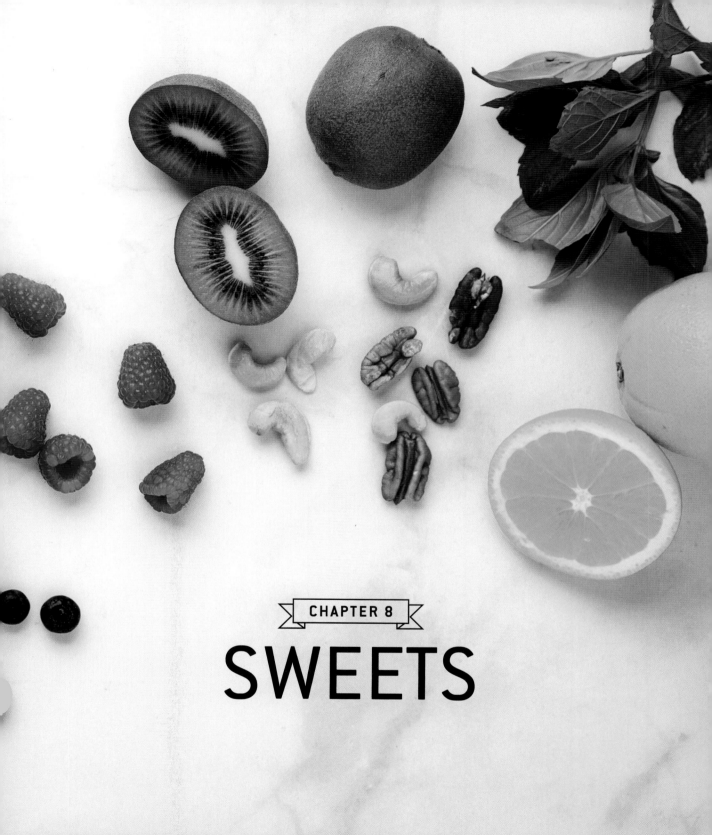

CHAPTER 8

SWEETS

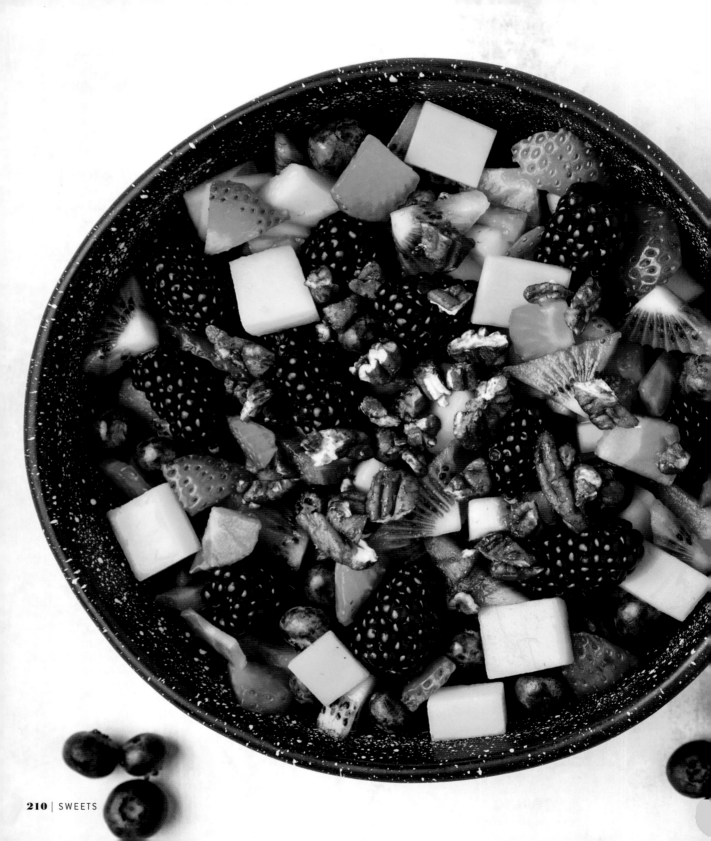

CINNAMON-PECAN FRUIT BOWL

PREP TIME: **10 MINUTES**
COOK TIME: **5 MINUTES**
YIELD: **2 SERVINGS**

INGREDIENTS

¼ cup chopped pecans

½ tsp molasses

¼ tsp ground cinnamon

⅛ tsp cayenne

½ cup chopped mango

½ cup chopped kiwi

½ cup blueberries

½ cup sliced strawberries

½ cup blackberries

½ tsp freshly squeezed lemon juice (optional)

We bring home big fruit hauls and often make this dish to use up the uber-ripe fruit while it's fresh. Most of these fruits are available in bulk at warehouse stores, and you can use any fruit you have on hand. What makes this recipe special is the delicious, spicy, candied-pecan topping. We make a game of ensuring the last spoonful has some of each fruit and that final candied pecan.

1   Heat a medium saucepan over medium-high heat. Once hot, toast the pecans for 1 to 2 minutes or until fragrant. Remove from the heat before they burn. In a medium bowl, toss the pecans with the molasses, sprinkle with cinnamon and cayenne, and stir to combine.

2   Place the fruit in a serving bowl and sprinkle with the spiced pecans. Drizzle with lemon juice, if using. Enjoy immediately.

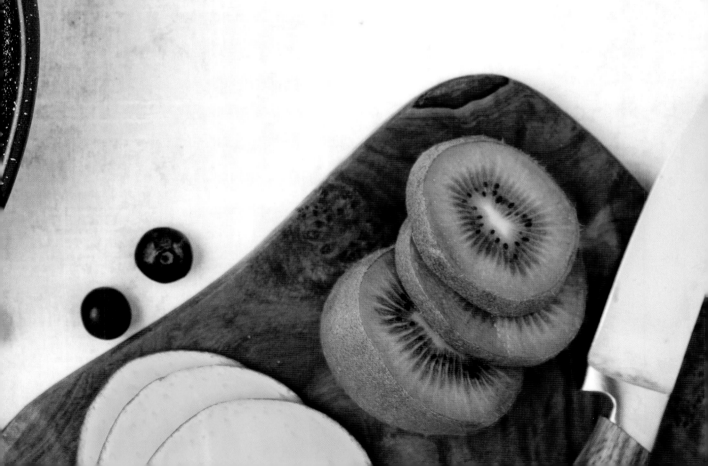

LIME-MINT PAPAYA AND JICAMA BOWL

PREP TIME: **15 MINUTES**
COOK TIME: **NONE**
YIELD: **1–2 SERVINGS**

INGREDIENTS

½ large papaya, thinly sliced (about 2 cups)

1 cup thinly sliced jicama

½ cup thinly sliced red onion

1 tbsp freshly squeezed lime juice

1 tsp apple cider vinegar

⅛ tsp cayenne, or more to taste

1 tsp minced fresh mint leaves

Lime wedges, to garnish

Is mint taking over your garden? Here is a way to fight back with a fork! Crunchy jicama compliments silky smooth papaya, while the red onion, lime, and mint combined with a dash of hot cayenne bring all the flavors to life. Too many people pass by these humble ingredients in the produce department. Grab a jicama next time you're shopping and give this sensational sweet a try.

1   Arrange the sliced papaya, jicama, and red onion in a serving bowl.

2   Drizzle with lime juice and vinegar and sprinkle with cayenne and mint. Adjust seasonings to taste and enjoy immediately.

✎ **NOTE:** You can opt to dice the papaya, jicama, and onion instead of thinly slicing them. Just be sure to keep the pieces uniform for optimal texture.

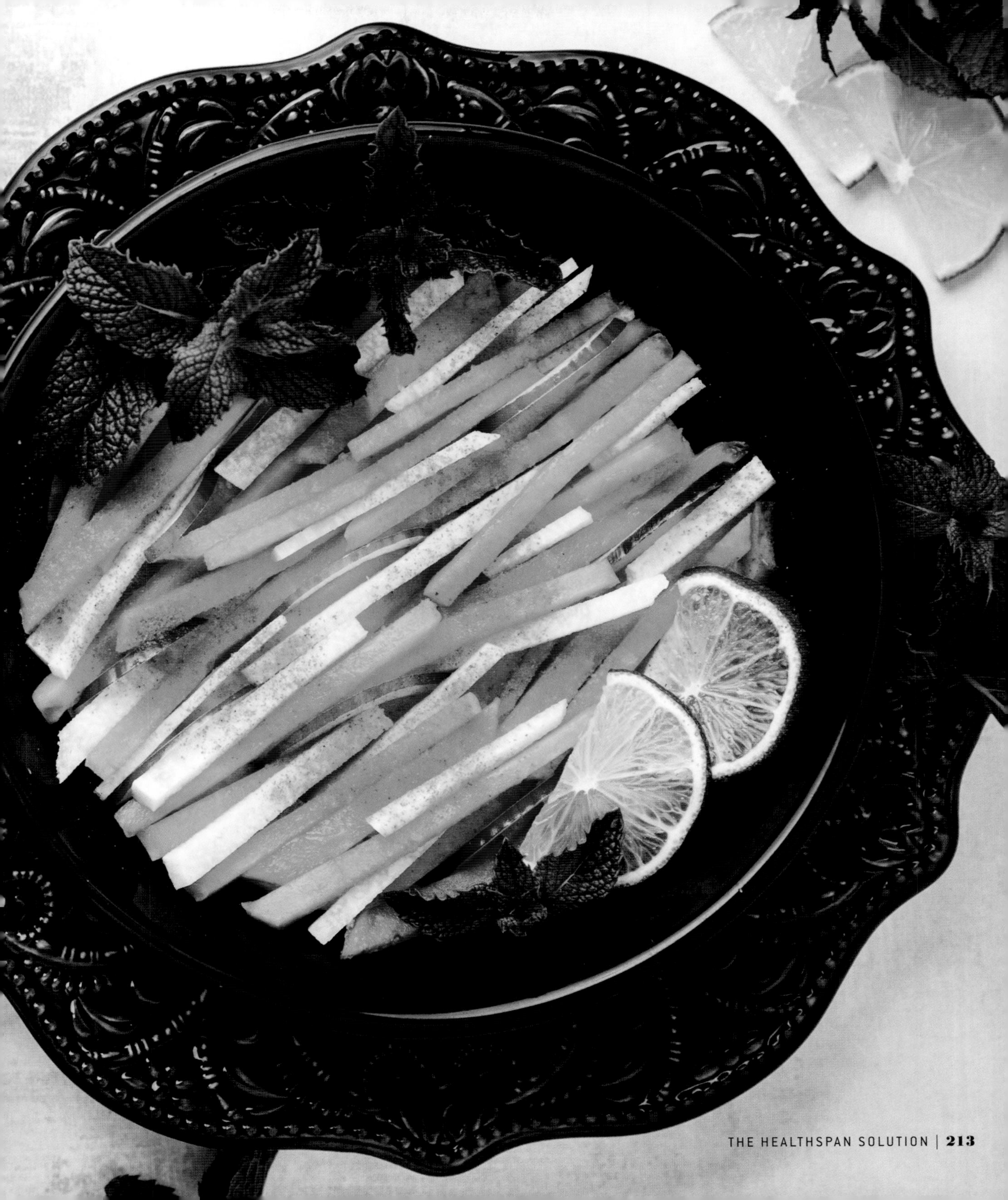

FRUSHI BOWL

PREP TIME: **10 MINUTES**
COOK TIME: **NONE**
YIELD: **1 SERVING**

INGREDIENTS

1 cup cooked black rice

1 tsp seasoned rice vinegar

1 cup diced mango

1 cup diced papaya

1 cup diced cucumber

1 tbsp nori strips or sprinkles,
   to garnish

1 tsp sesame seeds, to garnish

For the sauce

1 tbsp seasoned rice vinegar

2 tsp low-sodium tamari

1½–2 tsp wasabi powder or
   prepared wasabi

Fruit plus sushi? Frushi! While technically not *sushi* sushi, the rice, nori, and Japanese seasonings are certainly reminiscent of sushi. Sweet tropical fruits paired with toasted nori and drizzled with a salty, sapid sauce make this a special bowl you can savor.

1   Prepare the sauce. In a small bowl, stir together the vinegar, tamari, and wasabi powder.

2   Spread the rice in a large serving bowl and sprinkle with rice vinegar. Stir to combine.

3   Top with the mango, papaya, and cucumber chunks. Drizzle the sauce over the salad and garnish with nori and sesame seeds.

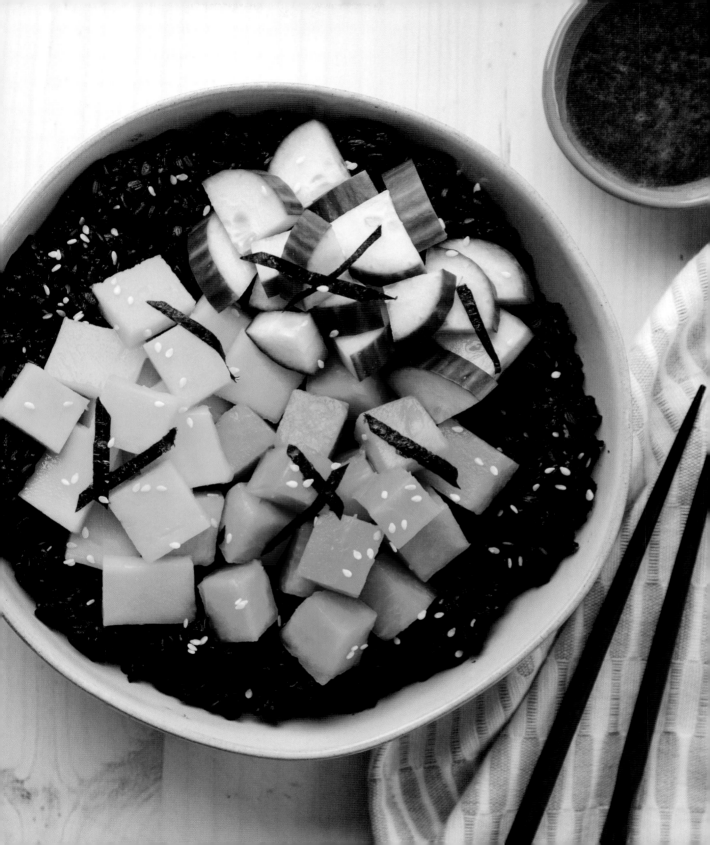

COCOA-MINT MIXED BERRIES

PREP TIME: **1 MINUTE**
COOK TIME: **5 MINUTES**
YIELD: **1 SERVING**

INGREDIENTS

3 cups mixed frozen berries

1 tbsp fresh mint chiffonade

1 tbsp chopped pecans

1 tsp cocoa powder

Because berries are bursting with powerful phytonutrients and many people love chocolate, why not entice you to enjoy more of these healthy gems with a magical sprinkle of cocoa (also a source of anti-inflammatory flavonoids)? We love stocking huge bags of frozen berries for use throughout the year for optimal affordability and a long shelf-life. Plus, they taste so comforting when warmed up in a big bowl.

1   Thaw and warm the berries in the microwave for about 4 minutes or heat in a small saucepan over medium heat on the stovetop for 5 to 7 minutes.

2   Transfer the berries to a serving bowl and top with the mint, pecans, and cocoa powder. Serve immediately.

✎   **NOTE:** You can also make this dish with fresh berries—just skip straight to step 2.

BASIL BERRY BLAST

PREP TIME: **5 MINUTES**
COOK TIME: **NONE**
YIELD: **1–2 SERVINGS**

INGREDIENTS

1 cup raspberries

1 cup blueberries

1 cup blackberries

¼ cup chopped black walnuts

1 tbsp molasses

⅛ tsp cayenne

1 tbsp basil chiffonade

Berries are considered one the best sources of bioactive compounds, such as phenolic acids, flavonoids, tannins, and ascorbic acid (vitamin C). These compounds have been shown to contribute to the myriad health benefits associated with berries, including reducing the risk of inflammation disorders, cardiovascular diseases, or various cancers. This batch of berries blasts your taste buds with a nice combo of tart, spicy, sweet, and aromatic, and also boasts an interestingly unique flavor.

1   Wash the berries and place in a medium bowl. Add the black walnuts and molasses and stir to coat.

2   Transfer to a serving bowl and sprinkle with cayenne (using more or less to taste) and basil.

CUCUMBER AND WATERMELON

with Fresh Lime and Mint

PREP TIME: **10 MINUTES**
COOK TIME: **NONE**
YIELD: **2 SERVINGS**

INGREDIENTS

2 cups chopped romaine lettuce
  or arugula

2 cups sliced cucumber, peeled and
  de-seeded

2 cups cubed watermelon

1 tbsp freshly squeezed lime juice

1 tbsp fresh mint chiffonade

Freshly ground black pepper,
  to taste

Sometimes, it's simplicity that brings out deep beauty. Here is a delightful way to celebrate summer melons, with just a squeeze of lime and dash of mint to round out the dish.

1 In a large serving bowl, plate the lettuce, cucumber, and watermelon. Drizzle with lime juice and sprinkle with mint and pepper. Enjoy immediately.

✎ **NOTE:** Basil is a delicious substitute for mint in this recipe.

KIWI, BERRIES, AND QUINOA

with Chili-Lime Sauce

PREP TIME: **10 MINUTES**
COOK TIME: **0 MINUTES**
YIELD: **4–6 SERVINGS**

INGREDIENTS

1 cup cooked quinoa, fully cooled

1 cup blueberries

1 cup sliced strawberries

1 cup diced kiwi

1 cup chopped romaine

1 tbsp basil chiffonade

For the dressing

2 tbsp freshly squeezed lime juice

2 tsp low-sodium tamari

1 tsp molasses or maple syrup

1 tsp hot 100% pure sesame chili oil

If you're not a salad person, then this dish is the one for you. It's a dessert and a meal in one big bowl. We've loaded it with kiwi and berries on a bed of crisp lettuce and then tossed in crunchy quinoa and a vibrant, punchy dressing. Feel free to amp up the heat if desired—sweet, tart, and spicy make a satisfying combination. This is a high-volume meal that's perfect for seasonal bulk fruit and vegetable purchases.

1 In a large bowl, combine the quinoa, fruit, and lettuce.

2 In a small bowl, stir together the dressing ingredients. Drizzle the sauce over the quinoa, fruit, and lettuce, and toss to combine. Garnish with fresh basil.

✎ **NOTE:** Toasted sesame oil can be used if heat isn't desired.

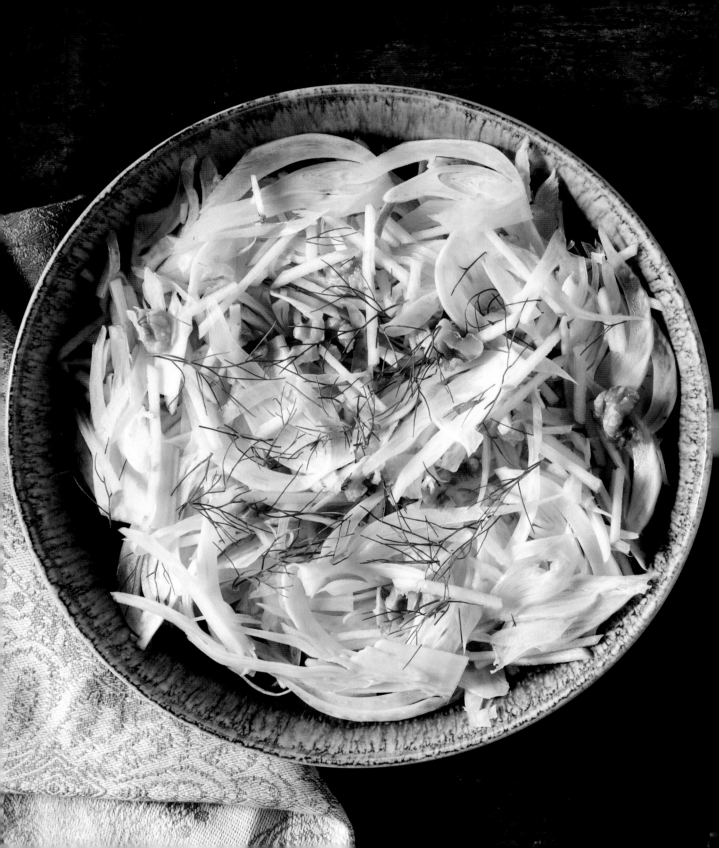

APPLE AND FENNEL
with Black Walnuts

PREP TIME: **15 MINUTES**
COOK TIME: **NONE**
YIELD: **2–4 SERVINGS**

INGREDIENTS

1 large fennel bulb

2 cups thinly sliced Granny Smith apple

2 cups thinly sliced Honeycrisp or Jazz apple

½ cup black walnut pieces

3–4 tbsp freshly squeezed lemon juice, to taste

Crisp, fresh fennel is often passed over in the produce bins, but it's a versatile vegetable with a salient anise flavoring. Together with sweet-and-tart apples as well as bold, earthy black walnuts, this salad is a crunchy, tasty, and wholesome bowl.

1 Cut off the fennel fronds close to the bulb, but reserve about ½ cup fennel fronds to add back into the salad. Cut the bulb in half and remove the core with two angled slices. Quarter the halves and thinly slice with a mandoline or knife.

2 Place the fennel, fennel fronds, apple, and black walnut pieces in a large serving bowl. Drizzle with lemon juice and toss to combine. Enjoy immediately.

✎ **NOTE:** You can add more or less lemon juice, depending on the sweetness of the apples.

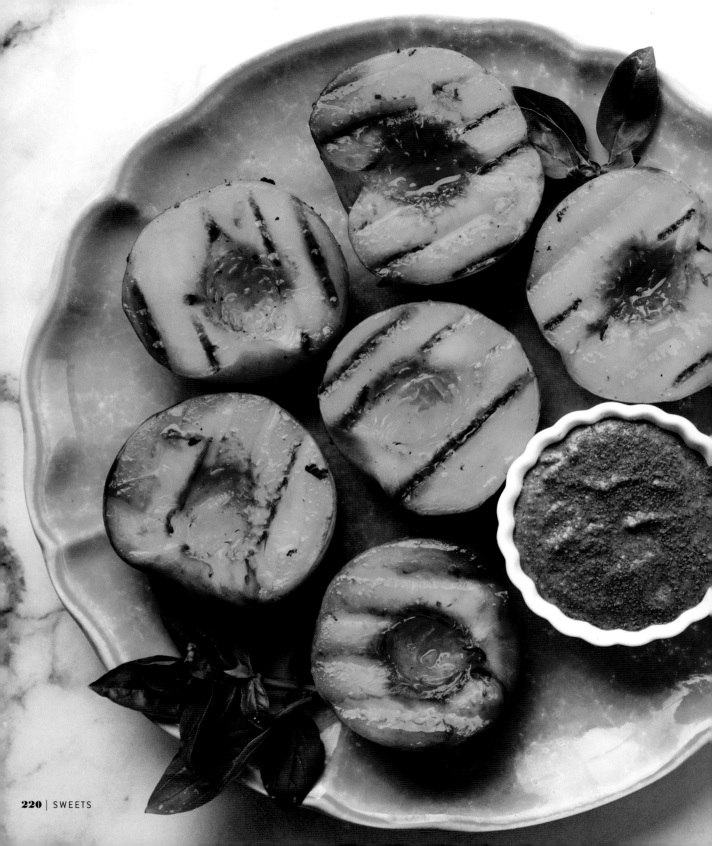

GRILLED PEACHES
with Basil-Cinnamon Cream Sauce

PREP TIME: **10 MINUTES**
COOK TIME: **10 MINUTES**
YIELD: **2–4 SERVINGS**

INGREDIENTS

4 peaches, halved and pitted

For the sauce

¼ cup Brazil nuts (or substitute raw cashews or hempseeds)

¼ cup unsweetened nondairy milk

1 Medjool date, pitted

1 tbsp fresh basil leaves (packed)

¼ tsp ground cinnamon

A sweet, creamy sauce with a basil-cinnamon kick is a delicious way to enjoy selenium-rich, cholesterol-lowering Brazil nuts, although cashews or hempseeds can easily be substituted here. The sweetness of summer peaches are enhanced on the grill via the caramelization process, making them an exquisite vehicle for this sauce.

1. Heat a cast iron grill pan over medium-high heat. Once hot, place the peach halves in the pan, cut side down, and cook for 5 to 10 minutes. Gently lift them off the pan with a spatula a couple of times during cooking to avoid sticking.

2. After 7 minutes, add ½ cup water to the pan, being careful to keep your hands clear of the rising steam. Allow the peaches to steam until the water has mostly evaporated. Continue to cook until the peaches feel warm to the touch and the skin begins to loosen.

3. In a blender, pulse the Brazil nuts until ground to a powder, but stop before they turn into a paste. Add the nondairy milk, date, basil, and cinnamon. Blend until smooth.

4. Remove the peaches from the heat. Transfer to a serving dish, drizzle with the cream sauce, and serve immediately.

✎ **NOTE:** To prepare the peaches on an outdoor grill, cook cut-side down over high heat for 4 to 5 minutes until grill marks appear. Flip over and cook until tender.

RED WINE AND COCOA PLUMS
with Cashew Cream Sauce

PREP TIME: **5 MINUTES**
COOK TIME: **10 MINUTES**
YIELD: **2 SERVINGS**

INGREDIENTS

4 medium plums, pitted and
   quartered

½ cup red wine

1 tbsp molasses

⅓ cup raw cashews

⅓ cup unsweetened nondairy milk

¼ tsp cocoa powder (optional)

Everything is better with chocolate and wine. Put them together and you have a magic combination. This dish is elegant and a surprisingly flavorful way to enjoy this vitamin C- and anthocyanin-rich stone fruit.

1 Heat a large saucepan over medium heat. Add the plums along with 2 tablespoons water and heat until they begin to caramelize, 3 to 5 minutes. Add the wine and molasses, stir, and cook until the sauce thickens, about 5 minutes more.

2 In a blender, pulse the cashews until they form a fine powder, but stop before they become a paste. Add the nondairy milk and blend until smooth.

3 Transfer the plums to a serving dish, drizzle with the cream sauce, and dust with cocoa powder, if using. Enjoy immediately.

✎ **NOTE:** You can remove the skins if they slip off while cooking (and you prefer not to eat them), but note that they are loaded with nutrients.

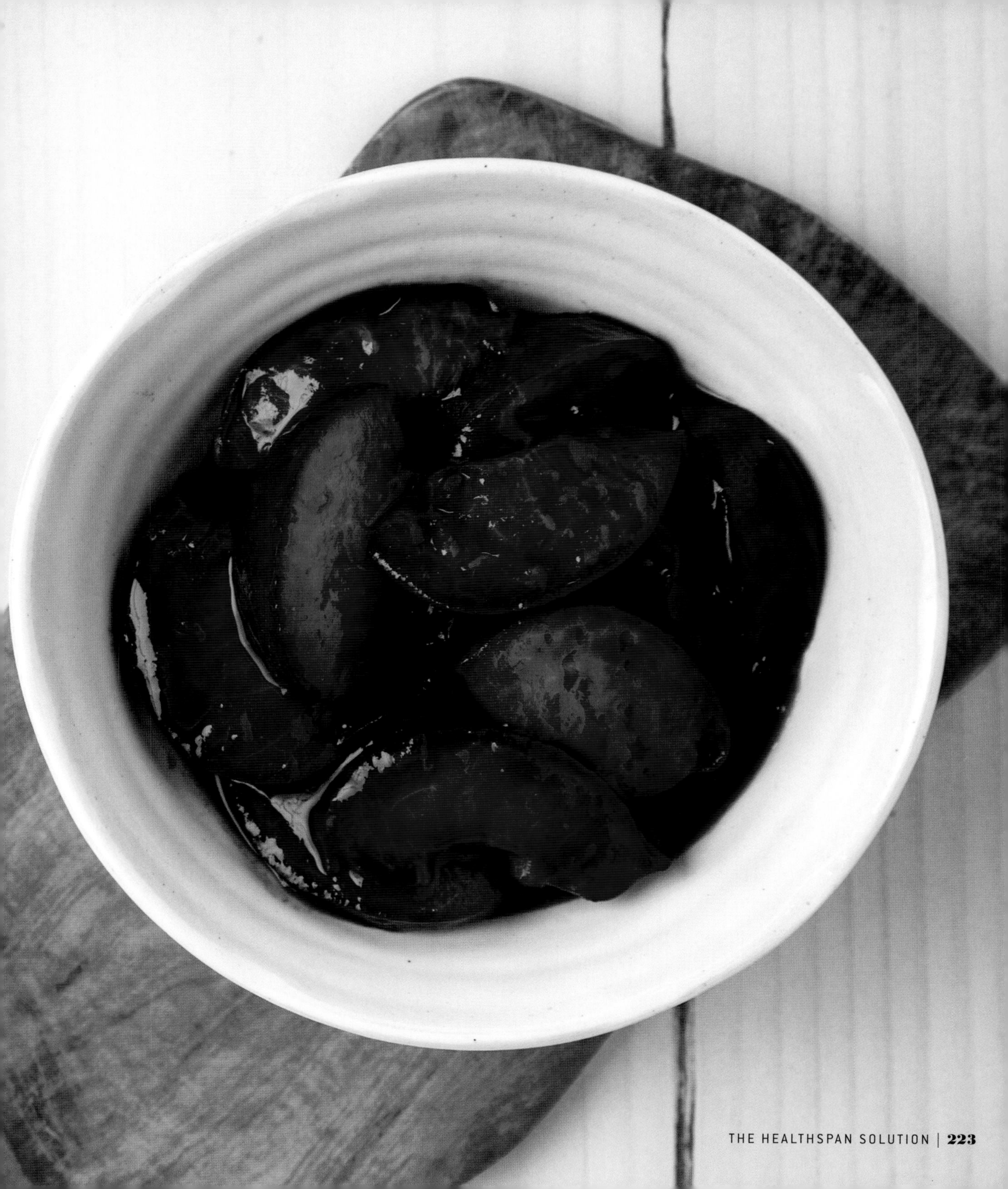

MIXED BERRIES

with Ginger-Mango Rhubarb Sauce

PREP TIME: **5 MINUTES**
COOK TIME: **5 MINUTES**
YIELD: **2 SERVINGS**

INGREDIENTS

2 cups chopped kale, stems
  removed

1 cup blueberries

1 cup raspberries

1 cup blackberries

1 cup sliced strawberries

¼ cup **Ginger-Mango Rhubarb
Sauce** (page 236)

Pinch ground cinnamon, to taste

Pinch ground cardamom, to taste

Our top-Triangle foods include stems, and rhubarb falls into that category. While it's common to balance this stem's notoriously tart flavor with sugar, we used mangoes and dates to create a scrumptious sauce. Poured over mixed berries and lightly steamed kale, and dusted with cardamom and cinnamon, it makes this dish pop with warm, complex flavors.

1 Heat a large saucepan over medium-high heat. Once hot, add the kale and 2 tablespoons water. Reduce heat, cover, and cook for 4 minutes, until the kale is wilted.

2 Place the kale in a serving bowl and top with the berries. Drizzle with the Ginger-Mango Rhubarb Sauce and sprinkle with cinnamon and cardamom.

✎ **NOTE:** Use less cardamom if you don't want the flavor to dominate, or if you don't like cardamom, omit.

ROASTED PLANTAINS

PREP TIME: **5 MINUTES**
COOK TIME: **25 MINUTES**
YIELD: **2–4 SERVINGS**

INGREDIENTS

4 equal-sized plantains

Options for topping

Allspice

Ground cardamom

Chili powder and lime juice

Cinnamon

Cocoa powder

Garam masala

Nutmeg

How many times have you walked by those green-looking "bananas" (plantains) and thought, "What do I do with them?" We're about to change that! These are easy to make and even easier to eat. It's the best of the banana flavor with just the right amount of sweetness. Once baked, the skin turns deep black and the starchy flavor becomes silky smooth and creamy, like a thick pudding. You can eat them plain or try some of the various toppings we've suggested. Be creative and have delicious fun.

1   Preheat the oven to 400°F. Line a baking sheet with a silicone baking mat or parchment paper. Place the plantains, whole, in their skin, onto the prepared baking sheet. Bake for 20 to 25 minutes, until the skins are completely black and they begin to seep juices. Remove from the oven.

2   To serve, peel one side and serve inside the skin, or remove the skin, slice, and plate. Top with your favorite seasonings or enjoy them on their own.

✎ **NOTE:** Select ripe plantains that are mostly black with some yellow spots, and flesh that is firm but yielding when pressed, like a ripe peach. It's best if all the plantains are similar in size for even cooking.

GRILLED WATERMELON, CUCUMBER, AND TOMATO

with Mint-Balsamic Drizzle

PREP TIME: **10 MINUTES**
COOK TIME: **20 MINUTES**
YIELD: **2–4 SERVINGS**

INGREDIENTS

1 small seedless watermelon

2 cups peeled, de-seeded, and sliced English (hothouse) cucumbers

3–4 medium vine-ripened tomatoes, sliced into wedges

2 tbsp thinly sliced fresh mint

1–2 tbsp balsamic vinegar, to taste

Freshly ground black pepper, to taste

Watermelon is one of the most abiding symbols of summer, and grilling transforms it magnificently, concentrating the flavors and adding an almost meaty texture with a hint of smokiness. Tossed with fresh cucumbers and tomatoes and topped with fresh mint and a drizzle of balsamic, this sweet is yet another reason to look forward to summer. Pile your plate high and take a long nap in a hammock afterward.

1   Cut the rind off the watermelon and slice into strips about 1 inch thick, 2 inches wide, and 5 inches long. (This will make it easier to grill.)

2   Heat a cast iron grill pan over high heat. Once hot, place the watermelon strips on the hot pan. Sear for 3 to 5 minutes or until grill marks appear. Flip the watermelon slices over and sear the opposite side for 3 to 5 minutes. (Typically, one side looks better.) Cut the seared watermelon into cubes. You will need about 3 cups watermelon for the salad.

3   Arrange the cucumber on a large plate and layer the watermelon and tomato on top. Top with mint, balsamic, and black pepper, to taste.

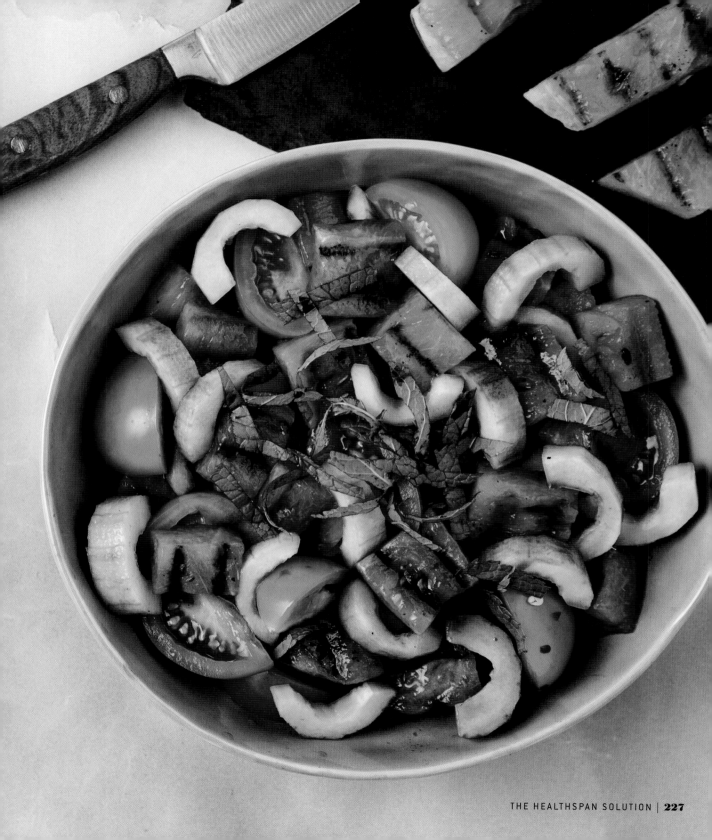

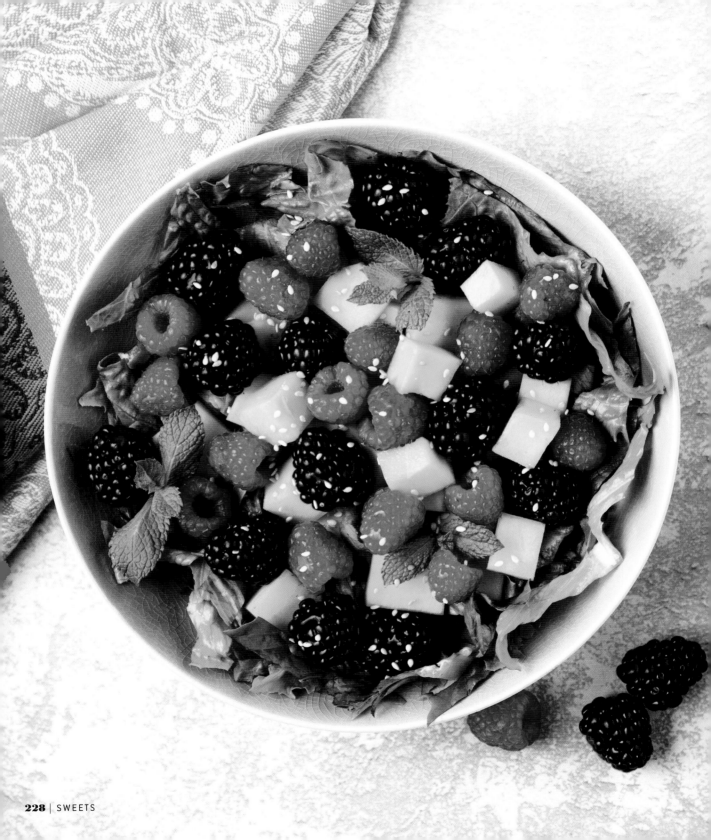

MANGO BERRY MINT BOWL
with Orange-Tahini Dressing

PREP TIME: **25 MINUTES**
COOK TIME: **NONE**
YIELD: **1–2 SERVINGS**

INGREDIENTS

1½ cups chopped romaine lettuce
   or arugula

1 cup chopped mango

½ cup blackberries

½ cup raspberries

1 tbsp chopped fresh mint

1 tsp toasted sesame seeds

For the dressing

1–2 clementines or small blood
   oranges (in season), peeled

1 tbsp tahini

½ tsp low-sodium tamari

2 tbsp balsamic vinegar

Blood oranges are a seasonal orange variety with crimson, anthocyanin-rich flesh and a berry accent to their citrus notes. Here, they are blended into a creamy tahini sauce that is drizzled over sweet mangoes and fresh berries for a unique and unforgettable dish.

1 Make the dressing. In a blender, combine the clementines or blood oranges, tahini, tamari, and balsamic vinegar. Blend until smooth.

2 Plate the lettuce in a serving bowl and top with approximately half the dressing. Then layer the mango, blackberries, and raspberries on top, and drizzle with the remaining dressing. Garnish with mint and sesame seeds, and serve immediately.

✎ **NOTE:** When blood oranges are not in season, clementines, tangerines, or oranges will work equally well in the dressing.

CHAPTER 9

SAUCES AND SEASONINGS

AVOCADO CILANTRO DRESSING

PREP TIME: **2 MINUTES**
COOK TIME: **NONE**
YIELD: **1 CUP**

INGREDIENTS

½ medium avocado

1 cup cilantro leaves

2 tbsp lime juice

1 tsp white miso paste

1 garlic clove

½ tsp chili powder

¼ tsp smoked paprika

¼ cup unsweetened nondairy milk (use to desired thickness)

The flavors of the Southwest and Latin America come together in a simple, creamy dressing that is perfect over salads and slaws or dolloped onto burritos, tacos, or cooked whole grains.

1   Using a standing blender, bullet blender, or immersion blender and a deep cup or jar, blend all of the ingredients for 30 to 60 seconds or until smooth.

2   Serve immediately or refrigerate in an airtight container for 2 to 3 days.

CARROT GINGER HEMPSEED DRESSING

PREP TIME: **5 MINUTES**
COOK TIME: **NONE**
YIELD: **1 CUP**

INGREDIENTS

¼ cup hempseeds

2 tbsp chopped fresh ginger

2 tbsp freshly squeezed lime juice

1 tbsp seasoned rice vinegar

½ tsp sesame oil

½ tsp white miso paste

1 tsp maple syrup

1 cup sliced carrots

This bright orange, vibrant dressing is almost a hippie cliche, but certainly a healthy and delicious sauce. Use it as a dressing or dip for fresh vegetables or over whole grains for a fresh, fun flavor festivity.

1   In a blender, pulse the hempseeds until ground to a powder, stopping before they become a paste, about 30 seconds. Add the remaining ingredients along with 3 tablespoons water, and blend until smooth.

2   This dressing is best served immediately but can be stored in an airtight container in the refrigerator for up to 3 days.

GREEN GODDESS DRESSING

PREP TIME: **5 MINUTES**
COOK TIME: **NONE**
YIELD: **1¼ CUPS**

INGREDIENTS

1 cup chopped fresh chives

1 cup chopped fresh parsley

2 garlic cloves

4 tbsp tahini

4 tbsp nutritional yeast

2 tbsp white miso paste

4 tbsp freshly squeezed lemon juice

1 tbsp chia seeds

A perfect play on a classic combination, thanks to Ray's mom, who is a master of plant-based cooking. Fantastically fresh, fragrant herbs lend a bright beautiful green hue, with zesty lemon and umami from miso and nutritional yeast balancing the flavors with hearty undertones. Double or triple the recipe to use throughout the week with your favorite veggies.

1   In a blender, add the chives, parsley, and garlic and blend for a few seconds. Add the tahini, nutritional yeast, miso paste, lemon juice, chia seeds, and ⅔ cup water, and blend until smooth.

2   Serve immediately or store in an airtight container in the refrigerator for 3 to 4 days.

✎ **NOTE:** If you are not using a high-powered blender, mince or chop the garlic before blending.

CREAMY CAESAR SALAD DRESSING

PREP TIME: **5 MINUTES**
COOK TIME: **NONE**
YIELD: **⅔ CUP**

INGREDIENTS

⅓ cup raw cashews

2 tbsp nutritional yeast

2 garlic-stuffed green olives (or 1 tbsp drained black olive slices)

1 tsp capers, drained

2 tsp anchovy-free Worcestershire sauce

2 tsp Dijon mustard

2 tbsp freshly squeezed lemon juice

¼ cup unsweetened nondairy milk

1 garlic clove

¾ tsp freshly ground black pepper

1 tsp nori flakes

As the briny, umami superstar of our Portobello Mushroom Caesar (page 163), this sassy dressing can also be enjoyed on any other salad or simply as an everyday, vivacious veggie dip.

1   In a blender, blend the cashews and nutritional yeast until ground but before turning into a paste, approximately 30 seconds. Add the remaining ingredients and blend until smooth.

2   Serve immediately or store in an airtight container in the refrigerator for up to 4 days.

LEMON BASIL DRESSING

PREP TIME: **2 MINUTES**
COOK TIME: **NONE**
YIELD: **1 CUP**

INGREDIENTS

½ cup chopped cucumber

1½ tbsp freshly squeezed lemon juice

¼ cup fresh basil, packed

1 Medjool date, pitted

1 tsp tahini

½ tsp low-sodium tamari

⅛ tsp roasted garlic powder

A light, refreshing dressing inspired by the Mediterranean and perfect over fresh fruit or salad greens.

1   In a small blender, add all the ingredients and blend until smooth.

2   Serve immediately or store in an airtight container in the refrigerator for up to 2 days.

POPPY SEED DRESSING

PREP TIME: **5 MINUTES**
COOK TIME: **NONE**
YIELD: **1¼ CUPS**

INGREDIENTS

1 tbsp chia seeds

¼ cup unsweetened nondairy milk

1 tbsp + ½ tsp apple cider vinegar

1 cup green grapes

1½ tsp Dijon mustard

2 tsp poppy seeds

This nutrified, whole-food variation of the classic poppy seed dressing is sweetened with white grapes and thickened with omega-3-rich chia seeds. Used in the Spinach Berry Salad (page 169), this easy dressing is a lovely complement to any fruit-based salad and can also serve as a dip or sandwich spread. Allow the chia seeds to thicken before adjusting the liquid to reach your desired consistency.

1   In a blender, grind the chia seeds into a powder. Add the nondairy milk, apple cider vinegar, grapes, mustard, and 2 tablespoons water and blend until smooth. Add the poppy seeds and stir to combine.

2   Serve immediately or store in an airtight container in the refrigerator for up to 3 days. Note this dressing thickens over time.

SWEET DIJON DRESSING

PREP TIME: **5 MINUTES**
COOK TIME: **NONE**
YIELD: **¾ CUP**

INGREDIENTS

¼ cup raw cashews

1 tbsp apple cider vinegar

1 tbsp sliced scallions, white and light green parts only

1 tbsp raisins or 1 Medjool date, pitted

2 tsp Dijon mustard

1 tsp low-sodium tamari

¼ tsp freshly ground black pepper

½ cup unsweetened nondairy milk

A dash of Dijon with a splash of sweet raisin makes this a simple, well-balanced creamy dressing. Tailored for the Roasted Cauliflower Salad (page 162), we have enjoyed this over other roasted veggies, salads, or cooked grains.

1 In a blender, pulse the cashews to a fine powder, but not all the way to a paste. Add the remaining ingredients and blend until smooth.

2 Enjoy immediately over the Roasted Cauliflower Salad, other salads, greens, cooked vegetables, or any dish that needs a sweet, creamy, tangy kick.

RANCH DRESSING

PREP TIME: **2 MINUTES**
COOK TIME: **NONE**
YIELD: **¾ CUP**

INGREDIENTS

½ cup raw cashews

¼ cup + 3 tbsp unsweetened nondairy milk

1¾ tsp apple cider vinegar

1 tsp freshly squeezed lemon juice

1 tsp minced flat-leaf (Italian) parsley

½ tsp low-sodium tamari

¼ tsp dried dill

¼ tsp freshly ground black pepper

⅛ tsp onion powder

⅛ tsp garlic powder

Ranch is one of the quintessential dressings to have on hand. This tangy, creamy, and absolutely decadent version is ideal to use with raw vegetables, potatoes, as a sandwich spread, over pizza, or pretty much anything. When in doubt, use ranch...especially this nutritious, fresh version.

1 In a blender, blend the cashews until ground but before turning into a paste, about 30 seconds. Add the remaining ingredients and blend until smooth.

2 Serve immediately or store in an airtight container in the refrigerator for up to 4 days.

GARLIC SAUCE

PREP TIME: **2 MINUTES**
COOK TIME: **3 MINUTES**
YIELD: **1 CUP**

INGREDIENTS

¼ cup raw cashews

2 tbsp nutritional yeast

¾ cup unsweetened nondairy milk

¼ cup light vinegar

2–3 garlic cloves

½-in cube fresh ginger

1–3 small Medjool dates, pitted

1 tsp arrowroot powder or
   cornstarch

A perfectly light sauce that lends the right amount of savory umami to any cooked dish.

1   In a blender, blend the cashews until ground to a powder, but stopping before they turn into a paste, approximately 30 seconds. Add the remaining ingredients and blend until smooth.

2   Transfer the sauce to a saucepan and heat over medium heat, stirring until it thickens. Pour over steamed vegetables or whole grains and serve warm.

✎   **NOTE:** If you are not using a high-powered blender, mince or chop the garlic and ginger before blending.

GINGER-MANGO RHUBARB SAUCE

PREP TIME: **10 MINUTES**
COOK TIME: **20 MINUTES**
YIELD: **5 CUPS**

INGREDIENTS

1 tbsp fresh ginger, minced

4 cups sliced rhubarb

2 cups sliced mangos

3 Medjool dates, pitted and chopped

Wondering what to do with those beautiful crimson stalks of rhubarb you see poking up each spring in the supermarket? Typically treated more as a fruit, rhubarb is technically a vegetable (opposite of the oft mistaken identities of the tomato, avocado, cucumber, and olive fruits being treated like vegetables). Enjoy this enigmatic stalk in this tangy, sweet, and unique combination.

1   Heat a large saucepan over medium-high heat. Once heated, place the ginger in the pan with 2 tablespoons water, until fragrant. Reduce heat to low, and add the rhubarb, mangos, and dates with an additional 2 tablespoons water. Cover and let simmer for 15 minutes. Turn off heat. Using an immersion blender, purée the mixture until smooth.

2   Serve immediately over fruit or greens, or store in an airtight container in the refrigerator for up to 5 days.

LEMON-TAHINI SAUCE

PREP TIME: **2 MINUTES**
COOK TIME: **NONE**
YIELD: **3 TABLESPOONS**

INGREDIENTS

2 tbsp tahini

1 tbsp freshly squeezed lemon juice

1 garlic clove, minced

Just a couple minutes, three ingredients, and a bit of water is all it takes to make this tangy, earthy, Middle Eastern staple sauce. Spread it on pita or serve it with falafel to bring a unique satisfying finish to your dish.

1   In a small bowl, combine all the ingredients along with 1 to 2 teaspoons warm water. Stir until smooth. Serve immediately.

SPICY PEANUT SAUCE

PREP TIME: **5 MINUTES**
COOK TIME: **20 MINUTES, IF ROASTING PEANUTS**
YIELD: **½ CUP**

INGREDIENTS

½ cup raw peanuts

2 tbsp rice wine vinegar

2 tbsp freshly squeezed lime juice

2 tsp minced fresh ginger

1 tbsp Sriracha or other hot sauce

1 tsp low-sodium tamari

1 tsp maple syrup (or mirin, a sweet rice wine)

Everyone needs a go-to peanut sauce recipe to have on hand for spring rolls, salads, noodles, and more. With a perfect peanuty balance of spicy, sour, salty, and sweet, this sauce makes everything taste amazing.

1   Preheat the oven to 350°F. Spread the peanuts on a baking sheet and roast for 20 minutes or until golden.

2   In a blender, process the roasted peanuts to a paste, 10 to 20 seconds. Add the remaining ingredients and blend until smooth.

3   Serve immediately, or refrigerate in an airtight container for 3 to 4 days.

✎ **NOTE:** To simplify this recipe, use ¼ cup unsweetened peanut butter in place of the roasted peanuts.

TOFU RICOTTA

PREP TIME: **10 MINUTES**
COOK TIME: **NONE**
YIELD: **2 CUPS**

INGREDIENTS

½ cup raw cashews

2 tbsp nutritional yeast

3 tbsp freshly squeezed lemon juice

1 tbsp apple cider vinegar

2 garlic cloves

1lb firm tofu, drained

2 tsp dried Italian seasoning blend

2–3 cups chopped kale (optional)

This plant-based stand-in for ricotta cheese is the filling for our delicious Eggplant Rollatini (page 175). It can also be used for stuffed shells, lasagna, as a salad topping, or anywhere else you might use ricotta.

1   In a blender, pulse the cashews and nutritional yeast until ground into a powder, but stopping before they become a paste. Add the lemon juice, apple cider vinegar, and garlic, and blend until a thick, creamy paste forms.

2   In a large bowl, crumble the tofu until it reaches a ricotta-like texture. Add the cashew mixture and the Italian seasoning to the tofu and use your hands to combine, taking care not to break up all of the tofu. Stir in the kale, if using, and mix until evenly combined. Refrigerate in an airtight container for up to 5 days.

UMAMI CHOCOLATE SPREAD

PREP TIME: **2 MINUTES**
COOK TIME: **NONE**
YIELD: **2 TABLESPOONS**

INGREDIENTS

1 tbsp tahini

1 tbsp molasses

½ tsp cocoa powder

⅛ tsp low-sodium tamari

An unexpected quartet of decadence. Luxuriously creamy and chocolatey, this is a silky spread for fruits, Roasted Plantains (page 225), breads, or anywhere else you feel inspired to use it.

1   In a small bowl, combine all the ingredients and stir. Enjoy immediately.

CHIPOTLE BUTTERNUT CHEESY SAUCE

PREP TIME: **10 MINUTES**
COOK TIME: **50 MINUTES**
YIELD: **2 CUPS**

This cheesy sauce can be poured over steamed or roasted vegetables, used as a soup base or pasta sauce, served as a topping for baked potatoes, or eaten with a spoon.

INGREDIENTS

1 small butternut squash

½ cup raw cashews

½ cup nutritional yeast

¾ cup unsweetened nondairy milk

2 tbsp freshly squeezed lemon juice

1 tbsp low-sodium tamari

½–¾ tsp ground chipotle powder

1   Preheat the oven to 375°F. Line a baking sheet with parchment paper or a silicone baking mat. Place the squash on the prepared baking sheet (whole) and roast until the skin is brown and bubbling, 20 to 40 minutes. Remove from the oven.

2   Once cool enough to handle, peel the squash, remove the seeds, and measure out 1½ cups roasted squash. (Remaining roasted squash can be transferred to an airtight container and refrigerated for a later use.)

3   In a blender, pulse the cashews and nutritional yeast until powdered, 10 to 20 seconds, stopping before they become a paste. Add the cooked squash, nondairy milk, lemon juice, tamari, and chipotle powder. Purée until smooth, about 60 seconds. Enjoy immediately, or store in the refrigerator in an airtight container for up to 1 week.

✎ **NOTE:** You can also use pre-chopped butternut squash, but cooking time will be decreased significantly depending on the size of the cubes, so monitor closely.

CASHEW PARMESAN SPRINKLE

PREP TIME: **10 MINUTES**
   PLUS 3 HOURS TO CHILL
COOK TIME: **NONE**
YIELD: **¾ CUP**

Grate these Parmesan-like sprinkles over food for an added burst of salty, umami goodness.

INGREDIENTS

½ cup raw cashews

¼ cup raw almonds

2 tsp nutritional yeast

1½ tsp freshly squeezed lemon juice

2 tsp white miso paste

2 tsp white vinegar

1   In a small food processor, place all the ingredients and pulse for 30 to 60 seconds until well combined. Scoop out the mixture and use your hands to form it into a thick disk, like a cheese wheel. Cover with plastic wrap and allow to chill for 3 to 4 hours.

2   Once chilled and firm, it can be grated like Parmesan for added umami flavor. Store in an airtight container in the refrigerator for up to 1 week.

EASY HOMEMADE BBQ SAUCE

PREP TIME: 5 MINUTES
COOK TIME: NONE
YIELD: 1½ CUPS

INGREDIENTS

1 (6oz) can tomato paste
2 Medjool dates, pitted and chopped
3 tbsp pineapple juice
1 tbsp molasses
2 tbsp low-sodium tamari
2 tbsp apple cider vinegar
2 tsp Dijon mustard
2 tsp freshly squeezed lemon juice
1 tsp freshly ground black pepper
1 tsp onion powder
½ tsp garlic powder
½ tsp ground chipotle powder
½ tsp smoked paprika
½ tsp liquid smoke
2 tsp tamarind concentrate (optional)

We gave the classic sweet, thick, tomato-based sauce a tangy edge and infused a whole lot of smoky heat. What makes this sauce special is that there is no cooking involved and the ingredients are easy to have on hand. Whip up a mess of this for the BBQ Chickpea Chopped Salad (page 164), use it in the Brunswick Stew (page 120), slather it on a Bean Burger (page 178), or use it as a marinade or dip. It's perfect for any dish that needs a punch of the smoky-sweet taste of the South.

1 In a blender, combine all the ingredients except the tamarind concentrate with 1 cup water and blend until smooth. Add the tamarind concentrate, if using, and stir to combine.

2 Serve immediately or refrigerate in an airtight container for 6 to 7 days.

✎ **NOTE:** For a spicy variation, use 3 teaspoons black pepper and 1 tablespoon tamarind concentrate.

ALABAMA WHITE SAUCE

PREP TIME: 5 MINUTES
COOK TIME: NONE
YIELD: 1 CUP

INGREDIENTS

¼ cup raw cashews
½ cup firm silken tofu
1 tbsp freshly squeezed lemon juice
1 tbsp prepared horseradish
2 tsp apple cider vinegar
1 tsp maple syrup
½ tsp Dijon mustard
½ tsp yellow mustard
1 tsp freshly ground black pepper
Pinch of kala namak (Himalayan black salt, see note)

You don't need an excuse to eat Alabama White Sauce. This signature sauce from Ray's hometown offers the right balance of creamy, peppery, mouthwatering goodness—y'all can use it as a spread, as a base for sauces or dressings, or however you prefer.

1 In a blender, pulse the cashews until ground to a powder but before turning into a paste, approximately 30 seconds. Add the remaining ingredients along with 1 tablespoon water and blend until smooth.

2 Serve as a dressing on the Deep South Bowl (page 150) or over cooked or raw vegetables, baked potatoes, cooked grains, tofu, seitan, or any other vehicle you would like to use to transport this classic sauce into your mouth. It will store in the refrigerator in an airtight container for up to 5 or 6 days.

✎ **NOTE:** Kala namak (Himalayan black salt) is a unique salt found in South Asia that contains sulfur and imparts an egg-like aroma and flavor. You can easily find this online and at many health food stores. You only need tiny amounts in recipes, so it will last in your pantry for quite a long time. You can substitute table salt here, but it will change the finished product.

GRANDMA MARIE'S TOMATO SAUCE

PREP TIME: **5 MINUTES**
COOK TIME: **1 HOUR 10 MINUTES**
YIELD: **5–6 CUPS**

INGREDIENTS

2 cups diced yellow onion

2 tsp robust olive oil

4 garlic cloves

1 (15oz) can tomato sauce

1 (28oz) can San Marzano
tomatoes, chopped

1 (6oz) can tomato paste

2 bay leaves

1 tbsp dried Italian seasoning blend

2 tsp sweet paprika

½ tsp freshly ground black pepper

¼ tsp ground fennel

¼ tsp crushed red pepper flakes

Ray's Sicilian Grandmother, Marie, is the inspiration for this classic sauce. His mother added her touch over the years and then he adjusted it with paprika, fennel, and pepper to capture the essence of the Italian sausage originally used to season. With the simplest ingredients, including those that can stay stocked in your pantry, this is a flavorful homemade sauce you can cook up and keep on hand to use over pasta, as a dipping sauce, or in the Eggplant Rollatini recipe (page 175).

1   Heat a large saucepan or Dutch oven over medium-high heat. Once hot, sauté the onions with as little water as possible, just enough to avoid burning, until they begin to brown, approximately 3 to 4 minutes. Add the oil in a small puddle in the center of the pan. Add the garlic and sauté for 30 to 60 seconds, or until the garlic is lightly browned, being careful not to scorch.

2   Add the tomato sauce, tomatoes, tomato paste plus 3 6oz-cans water, bay leaves, Italian seasoning, paprika, black pepper, fennel, and red pepper flakes. Bring to a boil. Once boiling, reduce heat, cover, and simmer 45 to 60 minutes, until thickened. If the sauce isn't thick, remove the lid and continue cooking uncovered for 5 to 10 minutes at the end.

3   Use immediately or allow to cool and then store in an airtight container for 3 to 4 days in the refrigerator or 1 to 2 months in the freezer.

MAYONNAISE

PREP TIME: **5 MINUTES**
COOK TIME: **NONE**
YIELD: **1 CUP**

INGREDIENTS

¼ cup raw cashews

½ cup extra-firm silken tofu

1 tbsp freshly squeezed lemon juice

1 tbsp seasoned rice vinegar

¾ tsp Dijon mustard

½ tsp apple cider vinegar

⅛ tsp kala namak (Himalayan black salt)

Rich, thick, and creamy mayo at your fingertips that is also better for your health than any store-bought option. Double or triple this recipe and keep it in your fridge at all times so you can make dressings, spreads, and sandwiches whenever the desire emerges.

1   In a blender, pulse the cashews until powdered, 10 to 20 seconds, stopping before a paste forms. Add the tofu, lemon juice, seasoned rice vinegar, Dijon mustard, apple cider vinegar, and kala namak. Blend until smooth.

2   Use immediately or store in the refrigerator in an airtight container for up to a week.

MAGIC MUSHROOM POWDER

PREP TIME: **5 MINUTES**
COOK TIME: **NONE**
YIELD: **4 CUPS**

INGREDIENTS

1 sheet nori, folded and cut into small strips

5oz dried shiitake mushrooms

1oz dried porcini mushrooms

2 tbsp roasted rice powder (see note)

1 tbsp toasted onion powder (see note)

1 tbsp garlic powder

Magically magnificent, this simple blend adds a striking impact. Blend up a large batch of this umami deliciousness, and divide it into small shakers. This will last a while and can be used to sprinkle a punch of umami savoriness to any dish.

1   In a high-speed blender, add the nori strips first, followed by the shiitake mushrooms, then the porcini mushrooms. Pulse a few times to get everything pulverized and then blend. Stop when the particles are finely ground, similar in texture to salt and pepper. (Grinding it too finely will make it a little messier and more difficult to handle).

2   Carefully transfer the mixture to a large bowl. Add the roasted rice powder, toasted onion powder, and garlic powder. Mix to combine.

✎   NOTE: Roasted rice powder and toasted onion powder are available in Asian specialty stores and from online retailers, such as Amazon.

MAGIC MUSHROOM GRAVY

PREP TIME: **10 MINUTES**
COOK TIME: **10 MINUTES**
YIELD: **3 CUPS**

INGREDIENTS

1 cup diced yellow onion

8oz gourmet mushroom blend, sliced

1½ cups **Simple Stock** (page 96) or low-sodium vegetable broth

2 tbsp nutritional yeast

2 tsp low-sodium tamari

1 tsp anchovy-free Worcestershire sauce

½ cup unsweetened nondairy milk

¼ tsp garlic powder

1 tbsp chopped fresh rosemary

1 tbsp chopped fresh thyme

½ tsp dry rubbed sage

2 tbsp cornstarch

½ tsp freshly squeezed lemon juice

We love this fragrant, savory gravy over potatoes of all kinds, whole grains, tofu, lentils, or even on its own. The not-so-secret ingredient that makes this gravy remarkable is the extra punch of umami that comes from the Magic Mushroom Powder.

1   Heat a large saucepan or Dutch oven over medium-high heat. Once hot, dry sauté the onions until they begin to brown, 2 to 3 minutes. Add 1 tablespoon water and the mushrooms, cover, and cook until the mushrooms release their liquid, about 2 minutes.

2   In a medium bowl, whisk together the broth, nutritional yeast, tamari, Worcestershire sauce, nondairy milk, and garlic powder. Add the mixture to the saucepan along with the rosemary, thyme, and rubbed sage. Reduce heat and simmer for 2 to 3 minutes.

3   In a small bowl, mix the cornstarch with 1 tablespoon cold water. Stir to make a slurry. Add to the saucepan and stir gently for 2 to 3 minutes until the gravy thickens. Add the lemon juice, stir to combine, and remove from heat.

4   Serve over Garlic Mashed Potatoes (page 180), on a plain baked potato, with whole grains, or over a heaping bed of greens.

TACO SEASONING

PREP TIME: **1 MINUTE**
COOK TIME: **NONE**
YIELD: **2 TABLESPOONS**

INGREDIENTS

1 tbsp chili powder

1 tsp ground cumin

½ tsp garlic powder

½ tsp onion powder

½ tsp dried Mexican oregano

½ tsp smoked paprika

This piquant, warm, and earthy salt-free blend can be used to season any taco filling, from rice and beans to roasted vegetables.

1   In a small bowl, combine all the ingredients and mix well. Use immediately, or transfer to a spice jar for storage.

FAJITA SEASONING

PREP TIME: **1 MINUTE**
COOK TIME: **NONE**
YIELD: **1½ TABLESPOONS**

INGREDIENTS

1 tsp chili powder

1 tsp paprika

1 tsp garlic powder

½ tsp onion powder

½ tsp ground cumin

½ tsp dried oregano

¼ tsp freshly ground black pepper

This is a slightly milder seasoning blend than our Taco Seasoning, but full of flavor and without the salt and sugar typically found in store-bought varieties.

1   In a small bowl, combine all the ingredients and mix well. Use immediately, or transfer to a spice jar for storage.

Endnotes

INTRODUCTION

1. Richard Wrangham and NancyLou Conklin-Brittain, "Cooking as a Biological Trait," *Comparative Biochemistry and Physiology Part A: Molecular & Integrative Physiology* 136, no. 1 (2003): 35–46.

CHAPTER 1

1. Eliza Acton, *Modern Cookery, in All Its Branches Reduced to a System of Easy Practice, For the Use of Private Families. In a Series of Receipts, Which Have Been Strictly Tested, and Are Given with the Most Minute Exactness* (London: Longman, Brown, Green, Longmans, and Roberts, 1858), viii–ix.

2. Wilbur Olin Atwater, "The Potential Energy of Food: The Chemistry of Food and Nutrition," *Century Magazine* 34, no. 3 (July 1887): 397–404.

3. Wilbur Olin Atwater, "Food and Diet," in *Yearbook of Department of Agriculture for 1894* (Washington, DC: US Government Printing Office, 1895), 367.

4. Wilbur Olin Atwater and Arthur Peyton Bryant, *The Chemical Composition of American Food Materials,* US Department of Agriculture Bulletin No. 28. (Washington, DC: US Government Printing Office, 1906).

5. Caroline Louisa Hunt, *School Lunches: Bills of Fare for Home and Basket Lunches, and for Meals Prepared at School,* US Department of Agriculture Farmer's Bulletin No. 712 (Washington, DC: US Government Printing Office, 1916).

6. Francis Adams, ed., *The Genuine Works of Hippocrates,* vol. 2 (London: The Sydenham Society, 1849): 703.

7. Atwater, *Food and Diet,* 368.

CHAPTER 2

1. World Health Organization and Annex B, "Tables of Health Statistics by Country, WHO Region and Globally," *World Health Statistics* (2016): 103–20, https://www.who.int/gho/publications/world_health_statistics/2016/EN_WHS2016_AnnexB.pdf?ua=1.

2. Hye Ryun Woo et al., "Plant Leaf Senescence and Death—Regulation by Multiple Layers of Control and Implications for Aging in General," *Journal of Cell Science* 126, no. 21 (2013): 4823–33.

3. Szymon Tomczyk et al., "Hydra, a Powerful Model for Aging Studies," *Invertebrate Reproduction & Development* 59, supp. 1 (2015): 11–16.

4. A. N. Khokhlov, "On the Immortal Hydra. Again," *Moscow University Biological Sciences Bulletin* 69, no. 4 (2014): 153–57.

5. Matt Kaeberlein, Mitch McVey, and Leonard Guarente, "Using Yeast to Discover the Fountain of Youth," *Science of Aging Knowledge Environment* (2001): pe1.

6. Luigi Fontana, Linda Partridge, and Valter D. Longo, "Extending Healthy Life Span—From Yeast to Humans," *Science* 328, no. 5976 (2010): 321–26.

7. Thomas B. L. Kirkwood, "Understanding the Odd Science of Aging," *Cell* 120, no. 4 (2005): 437–47.

8. Leonid A. Gavrilov and Natalia S. Gavrilova, "Evolutionary Theories of Aging and Longevity," *Scientific World Journal* 2 (2002): 339–56.

9. Konrad T. Howitz and David A. Sinclair, "Xenohormesis: Sensing the Chemical Cues of Other Species," *Cell* 133, no. 3 (2008): 387–91.

10. Dudley W. Lamming Jason G. Wood, and David A. Sinclair, "MicroReview: Small Molecules That Regulate Lifespan: Evidence for Xenohormesis," *Molecular Microbiology* 53, no. 4 (2004): 1003-1009.

11. Joseph A. Baur and David A. Sinclair, "What Is Xenohormesis?," *American Journal of Pharmacology and Toxicology* 3, no. 1 (2008): 152.

12. David A. Sinclair, "Toward a Unified Theory of Caloric Restriction and Longevity Regulation," *Mechanisms of Ageing and Development* 126, no. 9 (2005): 987–1002.

13. Carl M. McCay, Mary F. Crowell, and Lewis A. Maynard, "The Effect of Retarded Growth upon the Length of Life Span and Upon the Ultimate Body Size: One Figure," *Journal of Nutrition* 10, no. 1 (1935): 63–79.

14. Eva Bianconi et al., "An Estimation of the Number of Cells in the Human Body," *Annals of Human Biology* 40, no. 6 (2013): 463–71.

15. Ron Sender, Shai Fuchs, and Ron Milo, "Revised Estimates for the Number of Human and Bacteria Cells in the Body," *PLoS Biology* 14, no. 8 (2016): e1002533.

16. E. Cellarier et al. "Methionine Dependency and Cancer Treatment," *Cancer Treatment Reviews* 29, no. 6 (2003): 489–99.

17. Paul Cavuoto and Michael F. Fenech, "A Review of Methionine Dependency and the Role of Methionine Restriction in Cancer Growth Control and Life-Span Extension," *Cancer Treatment Reviews* 38, no. 6 (2012): 726–36.

18. F. Poirson-Bichat et al., "Growth of Methionine-Dependent Human Prostate Cancer (PC-3) Is Inhibited by Ethionine Combined with Methionine Starvation," *British Journal of Cancer* 75, no. 11 (1997): 1605.

19. David A. Sinclair and Leonard Guarente, "Small-Molecule Allosteric Activators of Sirtuins," *Annual Review of Pharmacology and Toxicology* 54 (2014): 363–80.

20. Elena A. Ponomarenko et al., "The Size of the Human Proteome: The Width and Depth," *International Journal of Analytical Chemistry* (2016): 1–6.

21. Brian K. Kennedy et al., "Mutation in the Silencing Gene S/R4 Can Delay Aging in S. cerevisiae," *Cell* 80, no. 3 (1995): 485–96.

22. Leonard Guarente, "Sirtuins, NAD+, Aging, and Disease: A Retrospective and Prospective Overview," *Introductory Review on Sirtuins in Biology, Aging, and Disease* (2018): 1–6.

23. Lamming, Wood, and Sinclair, "MicroReview," 1003–1009.

24. Dongryeol Ryu et al., "NAD+ Repletion Improves Muscle Function in Muscular Dystrophy and Counters Global PARylation," *Science Translational Medicine* 8, no. 361 (2016): 361ra139.

25. Jun Li et al., "A Conserved NAD+ Binding Pocket That Regulates Protein-Protein Interactions During Aging," *Science* 355, no. 6331 (2017): 1312–17.

26. Yujun Hou et al., "NAD+ Supplementation Normalizes Key Alzheimer's Features and DNA Damage Responses in a New AD Mouse Model with Introduced DNA Repair Deficiency," *Proceedings of the National Academy of Sciences* 115, no. 8 (2018): E1876–85.

27. Lindsay E. Wu and David A. Sinclair, "The Elusive NMN Transporter Is Found," *Nature Metabolism* 1, no. 1 (2019): 8.

28. Camilla Hoppe et al., "Differential Effects of Casein Versus Whey on Fasting Plasma Levels of Insulin, IGF-1 and IGF-1/IGFBP-3: Results from a Randomized 7-Day Supplementation Study in Prepubertal Boys," *European Journal of Clinical Nutrition* 63, no. 9 (2009): 1076.

29. Bodo C. Melnik, "Milk—The Promoter of Chronic Western Diseases," *Medical Hypotheses* 72, no. 6 (2009): 631–39.

30. Bodo Melnik, "Milk Consumption: Aggravating Factor of Acne and Promoter of Chronic Diseases of Western Societies," *Journal der Deutschen Dermatologischen Gesellschaft* 7, no. 4 (2009): 364–70.

31. Bodo C. Melnik and Gerd Schmitz, "Role of Insulin, Insulin-like Growth Factor-1, Hyperglycaemic Food and Milk Consumption in the Pathogenesis of Acne Vulgaris," Experimental Dermatology 18, no. 10 (2009): 833–41.

32. Bodo C. Melnik, Swen Malte John, and Gerd Schmitz, "Milk Is Not Just Food but Most Likely a Genetic Transfection System Activating mTORC1 Signaling for Postnatal Growth," *Nutrition Journal* 12, no. 1 (2013): 103.

33. Bodo C. Melnik, Swen Malte John, and Gerd Schmitz, "Over-stimulation of Insulin/IGF-1 Signaling by Western Diet May Promote Diseases of Civilization: Lessons Learnt from Laron Syndrome," *Nutrition & Metabolism* 8, no. 1 (2011): 41.

34. Zvi Laron and B. Klinger, "Laron Syndrome: Clinical Features, Molecular Pathology and Treatment," *Hormone Research in Paediatrics* 42, no. 4–5 (1994): 198–202.

35. Zvi Laron et al., "IGF-I Deficiency, Longevity and Cancer Protection of Patients with Laron Syndrome," *Mutation Research/Reviews in Mutation Research* 772 (2017): 123–33.

36. Sofiya Milman, Derek M. Huffman, and Nir Barzilai, "The Somatotropic Axis in Human Aging: Framework for the Current State of Knowledge and Future Research," *Cell Metabolism* 23, no. 6 (2016): 980–89.

37. Dan Buettner, *The Blue Zones: 9 Lessons for Living Longer from the People Who've Lived the Longest* (Boone, IA: National Geographic Books, 2012).

38. Michel Poulain, Anne Herm, and Gianni Pes, "The Blue Zones: Areas of Exceptional Longevity Around the World," *Vienna Yearbook of Population Research* 11, no. 1 (2013): 87.

39. Dan Buettner and Sam Skemp, "Blue Zones: Lessons from the World's Longest Lived," *American Journal of Lifestyle Medicine* 10, no. 5 (2016): 318–21.

40. Raymond J. Cronise, David A. Sinclair, and Andrew A. Bremer, "The 'Metabolic Winter' Hypothesis: A Cause of the Current Epidemics of Obesity and Cardiometabolic Disease," *Metabolic Syndrome and Related Disorders* 12, no. 7 (2014): 355–61.

41. Andrew R. Mendelsohn and James W. Larrick, "Sleep Facilitates Clearance of Metabolites from the Brain: Glymphatic Function in Aging and Neurodegenerative Diseases," *Rejuvenation Research* 16, no. 6 (2013): 518–23.

42. Valter D. Longo et al., "Interventions to Slow Aging in Humans: Are We Ready?," *Aging Cell* 14, no. 4 (2015): 497–510.

43. Gabriella Testa et al., "Calorie Restriction and Dietary Restriction Mimetics: A Strategy for Improving Healthy Aging and Longevity," *Current Pharmaceutical Design* 20, no. 18 (2014): 2950–77.

44. Julieanna Hever, *The Vegiterranean Diet: The New and Improved Mediterranean Eating Plan--with Deliciously Satisfying Vegan Recipes for Optimal Health* (London: Hachette UK, 2014).

45. D. C. Willcox et al., "Gender Gap in Healthspan and Life Expectancy in Okinawa: Health Behaviours," *Asian Journal of Gerontology and Geriatrics* 7 (2012): 49–58.

46. Natalia S. Gavrilova and Leonid A. Gavrilov, "Comments on Dietary Restriction, Okinawa Diet and Longevity," *Gerontology* 58, no. 3 (2012): 221–23.

47. Bradley J. Willcox et al., "Caloric Restriction, the Traditional Okinawan Diet, and Healthy Aging," *Annals of the New York Academy of Sciences* 1114, no. 1 (2007): 434–55.

48. Bradley J. Willcox and Donald Craig Willcox, "Caloric Restriction, CR Mimetics, and Healthy Aging in Okinawa: Controversies and Clinical Implications," *Current Opinion in Clinical Nutrition and Metabolic Care* 17, no. 1 (2014): 51.

49. Bradley J. Willcox, Donald Craig Willcox, and Makoto Suzuki, *The Okinawa Program: How the World's Longest-Lived People Achieve Everlasting Health—And How You Can Too* (New York: Harmony, 2002).

50. Donald Craig Willcox, Giovanni Scapagnini, and Bradley J. Willcox, "Healthy Aging Diets Other Than the Mediterranean: A Focus on the Okinawan Diet," *Mechanisms of Ageing and Development* 136 (2014): 148–62.

51. Gary E. Fraser and David J. Shavlik, "Ten Years of Life: Is It a Matter of Choice?," *Archives of Internal Medicine* 161, no. 13 (2001): 1645–52.

CHAPTER 3

1. Christopher J. L. Murray et al., "The State of US Health, 1990–2010: Burden of Diseases, Injuries, and Risk Factors," *JAMA* 310, no. 6 (2013): 591–606.

2. Ashkan Afshin et al., "Health Effects of Dietary Risks in 195 Countries, 1990–2017: A Systematic Analysis for the Global Burden of Disease Study 2017," *Lancet* 393, no. 10184 (2019): 1958–72.

3. World Health Organization, *The Double Burden of Malnutrition: Policy Brief,* No. WHO/NMH/NHD/17.3 (Geneva: World Health Organization, 2016).

4. Vesanto Melina, Winston Craig, and Susan Levin, "Position of the Academy of Nutrition and Dietetics: Vegetarian Diets," *Journal of the Academy of Nutrition and Dietetics* 116, no. 12 (2016): 1970–80.

5. Shelley McGuire, "Scientific Report of the 2015 Dietary Guidelines Advisory Committee. Washington, DC: US Departments of Agriculture and Health and Human Services, 2015," *Advances in Nutrition* 7, no. 1 (2016): 202–204.

6. Shelley Suter and Mark Lucock, "Xenohormesis: Applying Evolutionary Principles to Contemporary Health Issues," *Exploratory Research and Hypothesis in Medicine* 2, no. 4 (2017): 79–85.

7. W. Prout, "On Chemistry, Meteorology, and the Function of Digestion," *Gentleman's Magazine* (1834): 610–12.

8. Jennifer A. Woolfe and Susan V. Poats, *The Potato in the Human Diet* (Cambridge, UK: Cambridge University Press, 1987).

9. Julieanna Hever and Raymond J. Cronise, *Plant-Based Nutrition,* 2nd ed. (Indianapolis, IN: Penguin, 2018).

10. Janet C. King and Joanne L. Slavin, "White Potatoes, Human Health, and Dietary Guidance," *Advances in Nutrition* 4, no. 3 (2013): 393S–401S.

11. US Food and Drug Administration, "Final Determination Regarding Partially Hydrogenated Oils (Removing Trans Fat)," May 18, 2018, https://www.fda.gov/food/food-additives-petitions/final-determination-regarding-partially-hydrogenated-oils-removing-trans-fat.

12. Raymond J. Cronise, David A. Sinclair, and Andrew A. Bremer, "The 'Metabolic Winter' Hypothesis: A Cause of the Current Epidemics of Obesity and Cardiometabolic Disease," *Metabolic Syndrome and Related Disorders* 12, no. 7 (2014): 355–61.

13. Raymond J. Cronise, David A. Sinclair, and Andrew A. Bremer, "Oxidative Priority, Meal Frequency, and the Energy Economy of Food and Activity: Implications for Longevity, Obesity, and Cardiometabolic Disease," *Metabolic Syndrome and Related Disorders* 15, no. 1 (2017): 6–17.

14. Julieanna Hever and Raymond J. Cronise, "Plant-based Nutrition for Healthcare Professionals: Implementing Diet as a Primary Modality in the Prevention and Treatment of Chronic Disease," *Journal of Geriatric Cardiology* 14, no. 5 (2017): 355.

15. Masaru Teramoto and Timothy J. Bungum, "Mortality and Longevity of Elite Athletes," *Journal of Science and Medicine in Sport* 13, no. 4 (2010): 410–16.

16. Herbert W. Olson et al., "The Longevity and Morbidity of College Athletes," *Physician and Sportsmedicine* 6, no. 8 (1978): 62–65.

17. Cronise, Sinclair, and Bremer, "Oxidative Priority, Meal Frequency, and the Energy Economy of Food and Activity," 6–17.

18. Marc K. Hellerstein, "No Common Energy Currency: De Novo Lipogenesis as the Road Less Traveled," *American Journal of Clinical Nutrition* 74, no. 6 (2001): 707–708.

19. M. K. Hellerstein, "De Novo Lipogenesis in Humans: Metabolic and Regulatory Aspects," *European Journal of Clinical Nutrition* 53, no. s1 (1999): s53.

20. M. K. Hellerstein, M. Christiansen, S. Kaempfer, C. Kletke, K. Wu, J. S. Reid, K. Mulligan, N. S. Hellerstein, and C. H. Shackleton, "Measurement of De Novo Hepatic Lipogenesis in Humans Using Stable Isotopes," *Journal of Clinical Investigation* 87, no. 5 (1991): 1841–52.

21. Kevin J. Acheson, Y. Schutz, T. Bessard, J. P. Flatt, and E. Jequier, "Carbohydrate Metabolism and De Novo Lipogenesis in Human Obesity," *American Journal of Clinical Nutrition* 45, no. 1 (1987): 78–85.

22. Erik O. Diaz, Andrew M. Prentice, Gail R. Goldberg, P. R. Murgatroyd, and W. A. Coward, "Metabolic Response to Experimental Overfeeding in Lean and Overweight Healthy Volunteers," *American Journal of Clinical Nutrition* 56, no. 4 (1992): 641–55.

23. James O. Hill and Andrew M. Prentice, "Sugar and Body Weight Regulation," *American Journal of Clinical Nutrition* 62, no. 1 (1995): 264S–73S.

24. Regina M. McDevitt, Sarah J. Bott, Marilyn Harding, W. Andrew Coward, Leslie J. Bluck, and Andrew M. Prentice, "De Novo Lipogenesis During Controlled Overfeeding with Sucrose or Glucose in Lean and Obese Women," *American Journal of Clinical Nutrition* 74, no. 6 (2001): 737–46.

25. Robert Alexander McCance and Robert Daniel Lawrence, *The Carbohydrate Content of Foods* (London: H. M. Stationery Office, 1929).

26. Joanne Slavin, "Fiber and Prebiotics: Mechanisms and Health Benefits," *Nutrients* 5, no. 4 (2013): 1417–35.

27. Edward C. Deehan and Jens Walter, "The Fiber Gap and the Disappearing Gut Microbiome: Implications for Human Nutrition," *Trends in Endocrinology & Metabolism* 27, no. 5 (2016): 239–42.

28. Ron Sender, Shai Fuchs, and Ron Milo, "Revised Estimates for the Number of Human and Bacteria Cells in the Body," *PLoS Biology* 14, no. 8 (2016): e1002533.

29. Hannah D. Holscher, "Dietary Fiber and Prebiotics and the Gastrointestinal Microbiota," *Gut Microbes* 8, no. 2 (2017): 172–84.

30. Fan-Jhen Dai and Chi-Fai Chau, "Classification and Regulatory Perspectives of Dietary Fiber," *Journal of Food and Drug Analysis* 25, no. 1 (2017): 37–42.

31. Glenn R. Gibson et al., "Expert Consensus Document: The International Scientific Association for Probiotics and Prebiotics (ISAPP) Consensus Statement on the Definition and Scope of Prebiotics," *Nature Reviews Gastroenterology & Hepatology* 14, no. 8 (2017): 491.

32. Holscher, "Dietary Fiber and Prebiotics and the Gastrointestinal Microbiota," 172–84.

33. Gijs den Besten et al., "The Role of Short-Chain Fatty Acids in the Interplay Between Diet, Gut Microbiota, and Host Energy Metabolism," *Journal of Lipid Research* 54, no. 9 (2013): 2325–40.

34. Khawaja Muhammad Bashir and Jae-Suk Choi, "Clinical and Physiological Perspectives of β-glucans: The Past, Present, and Future," *International Journal of Molecular Sciences* 18, no. 9 (2017): 1906.

35. Claudia Lara-Espinoza et al., "Pectin and Pectin-based Composite Materials: Beyond Food Texture," *Molecules* 23, no. 4 (2018): 942.

36. Salima Minzanova et al., "Biological Activity and Pharmacological Application of Pectic Polysaccharides: A Review," *Polymers* 10, no. 12 (2018): 1407.

37. José Cruz-Rubio et al., "Trends in the Use of Plant Non-starch Polysaccharides Within Food, Dietary Supplements, and Pharmaceuticals: Beneficial Effects on Regulation and Wellbeing of the Intestinal Tract," *Scientia Pharmaceutica* 86, no. 4 (2018): 49.

38. J. L. Buttriss and C. S. Stokes, "Dietary Fibre and Health: An Overview," *Nutrition Bulletin* 33, no. 3 (2008): 186–200.

39. Diane F. Birt et al., "Resistant Starch: Promise for Improving Human Health," *Advances in Nutrition* 4, no. 6 (2013): 587–601.

40. Gertjan Schaafsma and Joanne L. Slavin, "Significance of Inulin Fructans in the Human Diet," *Comprehensive Reviews in Food Science and Food Safety* 14, no. 1 (2015): 37–47.

41. Shuruq Almodaifer et al., "Role of Phytochemicals in Health and Nutrition," *BAOJ Nutrition* 3, no. 2 (2017): 028.

42. Alireza Milani et al., "Carotenoids: Biochemistry, Pharmacology and Treatment," *British Journal of Pharmacology* 174, no. 11 (2017): 1290–1324.

43. Wilhelm Stahl and Helmut Sies, "β-Carotene and Other Carotenoids in Protection from Sunlight," *American Journal of Clinical Nutrition* 96, no. 5 (2012): 1179S–84S.

44. A. N. Panche, A. D. Diwan, and S. R. Chandra, "Flavonoids: An Overview," *Journal of Nutritional Science* 5 (2016): e47.

45. Asif Ahmad et al., "Mechanisms Involved in the Therapeutic Effects of Soybean (Glycine Max)," *International Journal of Food Properties* 17, no. 6 (2014): 1332–54.

46. Donald Craig Willcox, Giovanni Scapagnini, and Bradley J. Willcox, "Healthy Aging Diets Other Than the Mediterranean: A Focus on the Okinawan Diet," *Mechanisms of Ageing and Development* 136 (2014): 148–62.

47. A. Speciale et al., "Nutritional Antioxidants and Adaptive Cell Responses: An Update," *Current Molecular Medicine* 11, no. 9 (2011): 770–89.

48. Yiwei Li et al., "Regulation of Akt/FOXO3a/GSK-3β/AR Signaling Network by Isoflavone in Prostate Cancer Cells," *Journal of Biological Chemistry* 283, no. 41 (2008): 27707–16.

49. Susan Hewlings and Douglas Kalman, "Curcumin: A Review of Its Effects on Human Health," *Foods* 6, no. 10 (2017): 92.

50. Farrell Frankel et al., "Health Functionality of Organosulfides: A Review," *International Journal of Food Properties* 19, no. 3 (2016): 537–48.

51. Pablo F. Cavagnaro et al., "Effect of Cooking on Garlic (Allium sativum L.) Antiplatelet Activity and Thiosulfinates Content," *Journal of Agricultural and Food Chemistry* 55, no. 4 (2007): 1280–88.

52. Francisco J. Barba et al., "Bioavailability of Glucosinolates and Their Breakdown Products: Impact of Processing," *Frontiers in Nutrition* 3 (2016): 24.

53. Anika Eva Wagner, Anna Maria Terschluesen, and Gerald Rimbach, "Health Promoting Effects of Brassica-derived Phytochemicals: From Chemopreventive and Anti-inflammatory Activities to Epigenetic Regulation," *Oxidative Medicine and Cellular Longevity* (2013): 964539.

54. Sameer Khalil Ghawi, Lisa Methven, and Keshavan Niranjan, "The Potential to Intensify Sulforaphane Formation in Cooked Broccoli (Brassica oleracea var. Italica) Using Mustard Seeds (Sinapis alba)," *Food Chemistry* 138, no. 2–3 (2013): 1734–41.

55. Edward B. Dosz and Elizabeth H. Jeffery, "Modifying the Processing and Handling of Frozen Broccoli for Increased Sulforaphane Formation," *Journal of Food Science* 78, no. 9 (2013): H1459–63.

56. David J. A. Jenkins et al., "Effects of a Dietary Portfolio of Cholesterol-lowering Foods vs Lovastatin on Serum Lipids and C-reactive Protein," *JAMA* 290, no. 4 (2003): 502–10.

57. David J. A. Jenkins et al., "Direct Comparison of a Dietary Portfolio of Cholesterol-lowering Foods with a Statin in Hypercholesterolemic Participants," *American Journal of Clinical Nutrition* 81, no. 2 (2005): 380–87.

58. David J. A. Jenkins et al., "Assessment of the Longer-term Effects of a Dietary Portfolio of Cholesterol-lowering Foods in Hypercholesterolemia," *American Journal of Clinical Nutrition* 83, no. 3 (2006): 582–91.

59. Alvin Berger, Peter J. H. Jones, and Suhad S. Abumweis, "Plant Sterols: Factors Affecting Their Efficacy and Safety as Functional Food Ingredients," *Lipids in Health and Disease* 3, no. 1 (2004): 5.

60. Min Jia et al., "Potential Antiosteoporotic Agents from Plants: A Comprehensive Review," *Evidence-Based Complementary and Alternative Medicine* (2012): 364604.

61. Susan M. Potter et al., "Soy Protein and Isoflavones: Their Effects on Blood Lipids and Bone Density in Postmenopausal Women," *American Journal of Clinical Nutrition* 68, no. 6 (1998): 1375S–79S.

62. National Institutes of Health, "Office of Dietary Supplements—Vitamin B12," November 29, 2018, https://ods.od.nih.gov/factsheets/VitaminB12-HealthProfessional/#h6.

63. Gianluca Rizzo et al., "Vitamin B12 Among Vegetarians: Status, Assessment and Supplementation," *Nutrients* 8, no. 12 (2016): 767.

64. N. Dali-Youcef, and E. Andres, "An Update on Cobalamin Deficiency in Adults," *QJM: An International Journal of Medicine* 102, no. 1 (2009): 17–28.

65. Ralph Carmel, "How I Treat Cobalamin (Vitamin B12) Deficiency," *Blood* 112, no. 6 (2008): 2214–21.

66. Sven R. Olson, Thomas G. Deloughery, and Jason A. Taylor, "Time to Abandon the Serum Cobalamin Level for Diagnosing Vitamin B12 Deficiency," *Blood* (2016): 2447.

67. Naveen R. Parva et al., "Prevalence of Vitamin D Deficiency and Associated Risk Factors in the US Population (2011–2012)," *Cureus* 10, no. 6 (2018): e2741.

68. Michael F. Holick, "The Vitamin D Epidemic and Its Health Consequences," *Journal of Nutrition* 135, no. 11 (2005): 2739S–48S.

69. Daniel E. Roth et al., "Global Prevalence and Disease Burden of Vitamin D Deficiency: A Roadmap for Action in Low☒ and Middle☒Income Countries," *Annals of the New York Academy of Sciences* 1430, no. 1 (2018): 44–79.

70. National Institutes of Health, *Vitamin D Fact Sheet for Health Professionals* (Bethesda, MD: National Institutes of Health, 2011).

71. Holick, "The Vitamin D Epidemic and Its Health Consequences," 2739S–48S.

72. David G. Hoel et al., "The Risks and Benefits of Sun Exposure 2016," *Dermato-Endocrinology* 8, no. 1 (2016): e1248325.

73. Fahad Alshahrani and Naji Aljohani, "Vitamin D: Deficiency, Sufficiency and Toxicity," *Nutrients* 5, no. 9 (2013): 3605–16.

74. Pornpoj Pramyothin and Michael F. Holick, "Vitamin D Supplementation: Guidelines and Evidence for Subclinical Deficiency," *Current Opinion in Gastroenterology* 28, no. 2 (2012): 139–50.

75. Goran Bjelakovic et al., "Vitamin D Supplementation for Prevention of Mortality in Adults," *Cochrane Database of Systematic Reviews* 1 (2014): CD007470.

76. Joline W. J. Beulens et al., "The Role of Menaquinones (Vitamin K 2) in Human Health," *British Journal of Nutrition* 110, no. 8 (2013): 1357–68.

77. Barbara Walther and Magali Chollet, "Menaquinones, Bacteria, and Foods: Vitamin K2 in the Diet," Vitamin K2—Vital for Health and Wellbeing, IntechOpen, 2017.

78. National Institutes of Health, "Office of Dietary Supplements—Vitamin K," September 26, 2018, https://ods.od.nih.gov/factsheets/VitaminK-HealthProfessional/#h2.

79. Maurice Halder et al., "Vitamin K: Double Bonds Beyond Coagulation Insights into Differences Between Vitamin K1 and K2 in Health and Disease," *International Journal of Molecular Sciences* 20, no. 4 (2019): 896.

80. Johanna M. Geleijnse et al., "Dietary Intake of Menaquinone Is Associated with a Reduced Risk of Coronary Heart Disease: The Rotterdam Study," *Journal of Nutrition* 134, no. 11 (2004): 3100–105.

81. Joline W. J. Beulens et al., "High Dietary Menaquinone Intake Is Associated with Reduced Coronary Calcification," *Atherosclerosis* 203, no. 2 (2009): 489–93.

82. Halder, "Vitamin K: Double Bonds Beyond Coagulation Insights into Differences Between Vitamin K1 and K2 in Health and Disease," 896.

83. Robin J. Marles, Amy L. Roe, and Hellen A. Oketch-Rabah, "US Pharmacopeial Convention Safety Evaluation of Menaquinone-7, a Form of Vitamin K," *Nutrition Reviews* 75, no. 7 (2017): 553–78.

84. Tai Sheng Yeh, Nu Hui Hung, and Tzu Chun Lin, "Analysis of Iodine Content in Seaweed by GC-ECD and Estimation of Iodine Intake," *Journal of Food and Drug Analysis* 22, no. 2 (2014): 189–96.

85. National Institutes of Health, "Office of Dietary Supplements—Iodine," September 26, 2018, https://ods.od.nih.gov/factsheets/Iodine-HealthProfessional/.

86. Angela Leung, Lewis Braverman, and Elizabeth Pearce, "History of US Iodine Fortification and Supplementation," *Nutrients* 4, no. 11 (2012): 1740–46.

87. Bruno De Benoist et al., "Iodine Deficiency in 2007: Global Progress Since 2003," *Food and Nutrition Bulletin* 29, no. 3 (2008): 195–202.

88. World Health Organization, *Assessment of Iodine Deficiency Disorders and Monitoring Their Elimination: A Guide for Programme Managers* (Geneva: World Health Organization, 2007).

89. National Institutes of Health, "Office of Dietary Supplements—Iodine."

90. Meika Foster et al., "Effect of Vegetarian Diets on Zinc Status: A Systematic Review and Meta-analysis of Studies in Humans," *Journal of the Science of Food and Agriculture* 93, no. 10 (2013): 2362–71.

91. Melina, Craig, and Levin, "Position of the Academy of Nutrition and Dietetics: Vegetarian Diets," 1970–80.

92. Elizabethe Cristina Borsonelo and José Carlos Fernandes Galduróz, "The Role of Polyunsaturated Fatty Acids (PUFAs) in Development, Aging and Substance Abuse Disorders: Review and Propositions," *Prostaglandins, Leukotrienes and Essential Fatty Acids* 78, no. 4–5 (2008): 237–45.

93. Barbara Sarter et al., "Blood Docosahexaenoic Acid and Eicosapentaenoic Acid in Vegans: Associations with Age and Gender and Effects of an Algal-derived Omega-3 Fatty Acid Supplement," *Clinical Nutrition* 34, no. 2 (2015): 212–18.

94. Tanya L. Blasbalg et al., "Changes in Consumption of Omega-3 and Omega-6 Fatty Acids in the United States During the 20th Century," *American Journal of Clinical Nutrition* 93, no. 5 (2011): 950–62.

95. Bradley P. Ander et al., "Polyunsaturated Fatty Acids and Their Effects on Cardiovascular Disease," *Experimental & Clinical Cardiology* 8, no. 4 (2003): 164.

96. Angela V. Saunders, Brenda C. Davis, and Manohar L. Garg, "Omega-3 Polyunsaturated Fatty Acids and Vegetarian Diets," *Medical Journal of Australia* 199 (2013): S22–S26.

97. José L. Domingo, "Nutrients and Chemical Pollutants in Fish and Shellfish: Balancing Health Benefits and Risks of Regular Fish Consumption," *Critical Reviews in Food Science and Nutrition* 56, no. 6 (2016): 979–88.

98. Food and Drug Administration, *Fish and Fishery Products Hazards and Controls Guidance* (Washington, DC: US Department of Health and Human Services Food and Drug Administration Center for Food Safety and Applied Nutrition, 2011).

99. Madeleine Smith et al., "Microplastics in Seafood and the Implications for Human Health," *Current Environmental Health Reports* 5, no. 3 (2018): 375–86.

100. Angelo Cagnacci et al., "Homeostatic Versus Circadian Effects of Melatonin on Core Body Temperature in Humans," *Journal of Biological Rhythms* 12, no. 6 (1997): 509–17.

101. D. X. Tan et al., "Significance and Application of Melatonin in the Regulation of Brown Adipose Tissue Metabolism: Relation to Human Obesity," *Obesity Reviews* 12, no. 3 (2011): 167–88.

102. Saul S. Gilbert et al., "Peripheral Heat Loss: A Predictor of the Hypothermic Response to Melatonin Administration in Young and Older Women," *Physiology & Behavior* 66, no. 2 (1999): 365–70.

103. Kurt Krauchi, Christian Cajochen, and Anna Wirz-Justice, "A Relationship Between Heat Loss and Sleepiness: Effects of Postural Change and Melatonin Administration," *Journal of Applied Physiology* 83.1 (1997): 134–39.

104. Scott S. Campbell and Roger J. Broughton, "Rapid Decline in Body Temperature Before Sleep: Fluffing the Physiological Pillow?," *Chronobiology International* 11, no. 2 (1994): 126–31.

105. Patricia J. Murphy and Scott S. Campbell, "Nighttime Drop in Body Temperature: A Physiological Trigger for Sleep Onset?," *Sleep* 20, no. 7 (1997): 505–11.

106. W. K. Stewart and Laura W. Fleming, "Features of a Successful Therapeutic Fast of 382 Days' Duration," *Postgraduate Medical Journal* 49, no. 569 (1973): 203–209.

107. Roberto Refinetti, *Circadian Physiology* (Boca Raton, FL: CRC Press, Taylor & Francis Group, 2016).

108. Corie Lok, "Vision Science: Seeing Without Seeing," *Nature News* 469, no. 7330 (2011): 284–85.

109. Conrad Schmoll et al., "The Role of Retinal Regulation of Sleep in Health and Disease," *Sleep Medicine Reviews* 15, no. 2 (2011): 107–13.

110. Mirjam Münch and Vivien Bromundt, "Light and Chronobiology: Implications for Health and Disease," *Dialogues in Clinical Neuroscience* 14, no. 4 (2012): 448.

111. Anna Alkozei et al., "Acute Exposure to Blue Wavelength Light During Memory Consolidation Improves Verbal Memory Performance," *PloS One* 12, no. 9 (2017): e0184884.

112. Megumi Hatori et al., "Global Rise of Potential Health Hazards Caused by Blue Light-induced Circadian Disruption in Modern Aging Societies," *NPJ Aging and Mechanisms of Disease* 3, no. 1 (2017): 9.

113. Eleonore Maury, Kathryn Moynihan Ramsey, and Joseph Bass, "Circadian Rhythms and Metabolic Syndrome: From Experimental Genetics to Human Disease," *Circulation Research* 106, no. 3 (2010): 447–62.

114. Martha Hansen et al., "The Impact of School Daily Schedule on Adolescent Sleep," *Pediatrics-English Edition* 115, no. 6 (2005): 1555–61.

115. Amy R. Wolfson and Mary A. Carskadon, "A Survey of Factors Influencing High School Start Times," *NASSP Bulletin* 89, no. 642 (2005): 47–66.

116. Kalena E. Cortes, Jesse Bricker, and Chris Rohlfs, "The Role of Specific Subjects in Education Production Functions: Evidence from Morning Classes in Chicago Public High Schools," *BE Journal of Economic Analysis & Policy* 12, no. 1 (2012): 1–34.

117. Lynne Lamberg, "High Schools Find Later Start Time Helps Students' Health and Performance," *JAMA* 301, no. 21 (2009): 2200–2201.

118. Judith A. Owens, Katherine Belon, and Patricia Moss, "Impact of Delaying School Start Time on Adolescent Sleep, Mood, and Behavior," *Archives of Pediatrics & Adolescent Medicine* 164, no. 7 (2010): 608–14.

119. Brittney Jung–Hynes, Russel J. Reiter, and Nihal Ahmad, "Sirtuins, Melatonin and Circadian Rhythms: Building a Bridge Between Aging and Cancer," *Journal of Pineal Research* 48, no. 1 (2010): 9–19.

120. Shin-ichiro Imai and Leonard Guarente, "NAD+ and Sirtuins in Aging and Disease," *Trends in Cell Biology* 24, no. 8 (2014): 464–71.

121. Anita Jagota, Neelesh Babu Thummadi, and Kowshik Kukkemane, "Circadian Regulation of Hormesis for Health and Longevity," in *The Science of Hormesis in Health and Longevity*, eds. Suresh I. S. Rattan and Marios Kyriazi (London: Elsevier, Academic Press, 2019), 223–33.

122. Pontus Boström et al., "A PGC1-⊠-dependent Myokine That Drives Brown-Fat-like Development of White Fat and Thermogenesis," *Nature* 481, no. 7382 (2012): 463.

123. Shin-ichiro Imai and Jun Yoshino, "The Importance of NAMPT/NAD/SIRT1 in the Systemic Regulation of Metabolism and Ageing," *Diabetes, Obesity and Metabolism* 15, no. s3 (2013): 26–33.

124. Ana P. Gomes et al., "Declining NAD+ Induces a Pseudohypoxic State Disrupting Nuclear-Mitochondrial Communication During Aging," *Cell* 155, no. 7 (2013): 1624–38.

125. Joseph T. Rodgers et al., "Metabolic Adaptations Through the PGC⊠1α and SIRT1 Pathways," *FEBS Letters* 582, no. 1 (2008): 46–53.

126. Sander L. J. Wijers et al., "Human Skeletal Muscle Mitochondrial Uncoupling Is Associated with Cold Induced Adaptive Thermogenesis," *PloS One* 3, no. 3 (2008): e1777.

127. Rodgers, "Metabolic Adaptations Through the PGC⊠1α and SIRT1 Pathways," 46–53.

128. Edward P. Weiss et al., "Effects of Matched Weight Loss from Calorie Restriction, Exercise, or Both on Cardiovascular Disease Risk Factors: A Randomized Intervention Trial," *American Journal of Clinical Nutrition* 104, no. 3 (2016): 576–86.

CHAPTER 4

1. Jayaram Chandrashekar et al., "The Receptors and Cells for Mammalian Taste," *Nature* 444, no. 7117 (2006): 288.

2. George H. Perry et al., "Diet and the Evolution of Human Amylase Gene Copy Number Variation," *Nature Genetics* 39, no. 10 (2007): 1256.

3. Shizuko Yamaguchi and Kumiko Ninomiya, "Umami and Food Palatability," *Journal of Nutrition* 130, no. 4 (2000): 921S–26S.

4. Eiichi Nakamura, "One Hundred Years Since the Discovery of the 'Umami' Taste from Seaweed Broth by Kikunae Ikeda, Who Transcended His Time," *Chemistry—An Asian Journal* 6, no. 7 (2011): 1659–63.

5. Kikunae Ikeda, "New Seasonings," *Chemical Senses* 27, no. 9 (2002): 847–49.

6. Kikunae Ikeda and Saburosuke Suzuki, Process of separating glutamic acid and other products of hydrolysis of albuminous substances from one another by electrolysis, US Patent No. 1,015,891, filed January 30, 1912.

7. Kenzo Kurihara, "Glutamate: From Discovery as a Food Flavor to Role as a Basic Taste (Umami)," *American Journal of Clinical Nutrition* 90, no. 3 (2009): 719S–22S.

8. Toshihide Nishimura and Hiromichi Kato, "Taste of Free Amino Acids and Peptides," *Food Reviews International* 4, no. 2 (1988): 175–94.

9. Juerg Solms, "Taste of Amino Acids, Peptides, and Proteins," *Journal of Agricultural and Food Chemistry* 17, no. 4 (1969): 686–88.

10. Carlo Agostoni et al., "Free Amino Acid Content in Standard Infant Formulas: Comparison with Human Milk," *Journal of the American College of Nutrition* 19, no. 4 (2000): 434–38.

11. R. H. Kwok, "Chinese-Restaurant Syndrome," *New England Journal of Medicine* 278, no. 14 (1968): 796.

12. Jennifer L. LeMesurier, "Uptaking Race: Genre, MSG, and Chinese Dinner," *Poroi* 12, no. 2 (2017): 7.

13. Anca Zanfirescu et al., "A Review of the Alleged Health Hazards of Monosodium Glutamate," *Comprehensive Reviews in Food Science and Food Safety* (2019), https://doi.org/10.1111/1541-4337.12448.

14. Lawrence H. Kushi et al., "American Cancer Society Guidelines on Nutrition and Physical Activity for Cancer Prevention: Reducing the Risk of Cancer with Healthy Food Choices and Physical Activity," *CA: A Cancer Journal for Clinicians* 62, no. 1 (2012): 30–67.

15. Alice H. Lichtenstein et al., "Diet and Lifestyle Recommendations Revision 2006: A Scientific Statement from the American Heart Association Nutrition Committee," *Circulation* 114, no. 1 (2006): 82–96.

16. Karen B. DeSalvo, Richard Olson, and Kellie O. Casavale, "Dietary Guidelines for Americans," *JAMA* 315, no. 5 (2016): 457–58.

17. Hayden Stewart et al., *The Cost of Satisfying Fruit and Vegetable Recommendations in the Dietary Guidelines*, No. 1475-2017-3876. (Washington, DC: US Department of Agriculture, 2016).

18. World Health Organization, "Increasing Fruit and Vegetable Consumption to Reduce the Risk of Noncommunicable Diseases," February 11, 2019, www.who.int/elena/titles/fruit_vegetables_ncds/en/.

19. Ashkan Afshin et al., "Health Effects of Dietary Risks in 195 Countries, 1990–2017: A Systematic Analysis for the Global Burden of Disease Study 2017," *Lancet* 393, no. 10184 (2019): 1958–72.

20. Dagfinn Aune et al., "Whole Grain Consumption and Risk of Cardiovascular Disease, Cancer, and All Cause and Cause Specific Mortality: Systematic Review and Dose-response Meta-analysis of Prospective Studies," *BMJ* 353 (2016): i2716.

21. B. Zhang et al., "Association of Whole Grain Intake with All-Cause, Cardiovascular, and Cancer Mortality: A Systematic Review and Dose–response Meta-analysis from Prospective Cohort Studies," *European Journal of Clinical Nutrition* 72, no. 1 (2018): 57.

22. Giuseppe Della Pepa et al., "Wholegrain Intake and Risk of Type 2 Diabetes: Evidence from Epidemiological and Intervention Studies," *Nutrients* 10, no. 9 (2018): 1288.

23. Dan Buettner and Sam Skemp, "Blue Zones: Lessons from the World's Longest Lived," *American Journal of Lifestyle Medicine* 10, no. 5 (2016): 318–21.

24. Stefano Marventano et al., "Legume Consumption and CVD Risk: A Systematic Review and Meta-analysis," *Public Health Nutrition* 20, no. 2 (2017): 245–54.

25. Rani Polak, Edward M. Phillips, and Amy Campbell, "Legumes: Health Benefits and Culinary Approaches to Increase Intake," *Clinical Diabetes* 33, no. 4 (2015): 198–205.

26. Xariss Sánchez-Chino et al., "Nutrient and Nonnutrient Components of Legumes, and Its Chemopreventive Activity: A Review," *Nutrition and Cancer* 67, no. 3 (2015): 401–410.

27. Megan A. McCrory et al., "Pulse Consumption, Satiety, and Weight Management," *Advances in Nutrition* 1, no. 1 (2010): 17–30.

28. Sandra Clark and Alison M. Duncan, "The Role of Pulses in Satiety, Food Intake and Body Weight Management," *Journal of Functional Foods* 38 (2017): 612–23.

29. Connie Weaver and Elizabeth T. Marr, "White Vegetables: A Forgotten Source of Nutrients: Purdue Roundtable Executive Summary," *Advances in Nutrition* 4, no. 3 (2013): 318S–26S.

30. Paul E. Stamets, "Notes on Nutritional Properties of Culinary-medicinal Mushrooms," *International Journal of Medicinal Mushrooms* 7, no. 1–2 (2005): 103–10.

31. Paul Stamets, *Growing Gourmet and Medicinal Mushrooms* (Berkeley, CA: Ten Speed Press, 2011).

32. Mary Jo Feeney, Amy Myrdal Miller, and Peter Roupas, "Mushrooms—Biologically Distinct and Nutritionally Unique: Exploring a 'Third Food Kingdom,'" *Nutrition Today* 49, no. 6 (2014): 301.

33. E. O'Neil, A. Nicklas, and Victor L. Fulgoni III, "Mushroom Intake Is Associated with Better Nutrient Intake and Diet Quality: 2001–2010 National Health and Nutrition Examination Survey," *Nutrition & Food Sciences* 3 (2013): 5.

34. Glenn Cardwell et al., "A Review of Mushrooms as a Potential Source of Dietary Vitamin D," *Nutrients* 10, no. 10 (2018): 1498.

35. Muthukumaran Jayachandran, Jianbo Xiao, and Baojun Xu, "A Critical Review on Health Promoting Benefits of Edible Mushrooms Through Gut Microbiota," *International Journal of Molecular Sciences* 18, no. 9 (2017): 1934.

36. Jiao-Jiao Zhang et al., "Bioactivities and Health Benefits of Mushrooms Mainly from China," *Molecules* 21, no. 7 (2016): 938.

37. Rávila de Souza et al., «Nuts and Human Health Outcomes: A Systematic Review,» *Nutrients* 9, no. 12 (2017): 1311.

38. Dagfinn Aune et al., "Nut Consumption and Risk of Cardiovascular Disease, Total Cancer, All-cause and Cause-specific Mortality: A Systematic Review and Dose-response Meta-analysis of Prospective Studies," *BMC Medicine* 14, no. 1 (2016): 207.

39. Effie Viguiliouk et al., "Effect of Tree Nuts on Glycemic Control in Diabetes: A Systematic Review and Meta-Analysis of Randomized Controlled Dietary Trials," *PloS One* 9, no. 7 (2014): e103376.

40. Jacqueline O'Brien et al., "Long-term Intake of Nuts in Relation to Cognitive Function in Older Women," *Journal of Nutrition, Health & Aging* 18, no. 5 (2014): 496–502.

41. Peter Pribis and Barbara Shukitt-Hale, "Cognition: The New Frontier for Nuts and Berries," *American Journal of Clinical Nutrition* 100, suppl. 1 (2014): 347S–52S.

42. Ujang Tinggi, "Selenium: Its Role as Antioxidant in Human Health," *Environmental Health and Preventive Medicine* 13, no. 2 (2008): 102.

43. Elisângela Colpo et al., "A Single Consumption of High Amounts of the Brazil Nuts Improves Lipid Profile of Healthy Volunteers," *Journal of Nutrition and Metabolism* (2013): 653185.

44. David J. A. Jenkins et al., "The Effect of Combining Plant Sterols, Soy Protein, Viscous Fibers, and Almonds in Treating Hypercholesterolemia," *Metabolism* 52, no. 11 (2003): 1478–83.

45. David J. A. Jenkins et al., "Assessment of the Longer-term Effects of a Dietary Portfolio of Cholesterol-Lowering Foods in Hypercholesterolemia," *American Journal of Clinical Nutrition* 83, no. 3 (2006): 582–91.

46. Melody J. Brown et al., "Carotenoid Bioavailability Is Higher from Salads Ingested with Full-fat Than with Fat-reduced Salad Dressings as Measured with Electrochemical Detection," *American Journal of Clinical Nutrition* 80, no. 2 (2004): 396–403.

47. Nuray Z. Unlu et al., "Carotenoid Absorption from Salad and Salsa by Humans Is Enhanced by the Addition of Avocado or Avocado Oil," *Journal of Nutrition* 135, no. 3 (2005): 431–36.

48. Ali A. Albahrani and Ronda F. Greaves, "Fat-soluble Vitamins: Clinical Indications and Current Challenges for Chromatographic Measurement," *Clinical Biochemist Reviews* 37, no. 1 (2016): 27.

49. Elizabeth Opara and Magali Chohan, "Culinary Herbs and Spices: Their Bioactive Properties, the Contribution of Polyphenols and the Challenges in Deducing Their True Health Benefits," *International Journal of Molecular Sciences* 15, no. 10 (2014): 19183–202.

50. K. Srinivasan, "Role of Spices Beyond Food Flavoring: Nutraceuticals with Multiple Health Effects," *Food Reviews International* 21, no. 2 (2005): 167–88.

Index

ACKNOWLEDGMENTS

Julieanna and Ray are grateful to Marilyn Allen, our magnificent agent, and our dedicated team at DK Publishing, especially Mike Sanders, Ann Barton, Jessica Lee, and the rest of the team for seeing and supporting our vision.

Thank you to our mentors and colleagues: Drs. David Sinclair, Andrew Bremer, Michael Greger, Dean Ornish, Maurice Blitz, Brian Iriye, Michael Klaper, and T. Colin Campbell. We appreciate the inspiration and support from these special people: Penn Jillette, Tim Jenison, Cyan Banister, Michael Potter, Marc Hodosh, Peter Diamandis, Dave Lakahni, Shale Martin, and Steve Davis. A loving hat tip to our support team at home: Dorene, Marty, Lois, and Renee.

Finally, we want to express sincere appreciation for our many followers, promoters, and supporters who are helping us transform 10,000 lives—you are THE reason we are here.

ABOUT THE AUTHORS

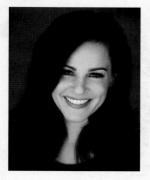

JULIEANNA HEVER, MS, RD, CPT, *The Plant-Based Dietitian*, has a BA in Theatre and an MS in Nutrition, bridging her biggest passions for food, presenting, and helping people. She has authored four books, including *Plant-Based Nutrition* (Idiot's Guides) and *The Vegiterranean Diet*, and two peer-reviewed journal articles on plant-based nutrition for healthcare professionals. She was the host of *What Would Julieanna Do?*, gave a TEDx talk, and instructed for the eCornell Plant-Based Nutrition Certification Program. She's appeared on *The Dr. Oz Show*, *Harry*, and *The Steve Harvey Show*. Julieanna is the co-founder and nutrition director for Efferos, and she speaks and consults with clients around the globe.

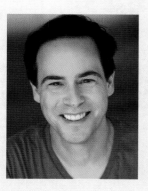

RAY CRONISE, BSc, is a scientist-innovator focused on diet and nutrition and the co-founder of Efferos, a lifestyle transformation company. He co-authored *Plant-Based Nutrition,* Second Edition (Idiot's Guides) with Julieanna Hever and is the mastermind behind Las Vegas magician Penn Jillette's plant-based diet 100-pound weight loss. A former NASA scientist and Matthew Kenney and Blue Lotus Culinary graduate, he's collaborating with leading academic researchers at institutions such as Harvard and the NIH to publish work at the intersection of healthspan and plant-based diets. He's been featured by *Wired Magazine*, TEDMED 2010, *The New York Times*, *ABC Nightline*, *The Atlantic*, *Men's Journal*, *The Guardian*, *Presto!: How I made 100 pounds magically disappear*, and *The 4-Hour Body*.